Nuclear Medicine Technology

Andrzej Moniuszko • Dharmesh Patel

Nuclear Medicine Technology Study Guide

A Technologist's Review for Passing
Board Exams

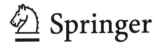 Springer

Andrzej Moniuszko, MD, CNMT,
ARRT(N), NCT, PET
Resurrection Medical Center
Chicago, IL, USA
mdandy52@yahoo.com

Dharmesh Patel, CNMT, ARRT(N)
Resurrection Medical Center
Chicago, IL, USA
deepatel82@gmail.com

ISBN 978-1-4419-9361-8   e-ISBN 978-1-4419-9362-5
DOI 10.1007/978-1-4419-9362-5
Springer New York Dordrecht Heidelberg London

Library of Congress Control Number: 2011929226

Printed on acid-free paper

Springer is part of Springer Science+Business Media (www.springer.com)

I would like to dedicate this work to my mother, Lila, who worked restlessly to ensure that her son had the opportunities never available to her, and to my daughters Beata, Marta, and Sabina for their unconditional love. I cannot thank them enough for their boundless affection, their indefatigable support, and the sacrifices they have made to make my life most rewarding. To Anna, for making me believe that anything is possible.

Andrzej Moniuszko, MD, CNMT, ARRT(N), NCT, PET

I would like to dedicate my work in this book to my sister Kanchan, my mother Kalavati, my father Lallu, and my cousins Nilesh and Dipesh for supporting me throughout the process of writing. It has been a great experience writing this book, which challenged my intellect at every step in the process.

Dharmesh Patel, CNMT, ARRT(N)

Preface

The Nuclear Medicine Technology Study guide is designed for technologists to serve as a practical tool to study multiple aspects of nuclear medicine. The book contains insights from the wide spectrum of nuclear medicine concepts and principles, providing an array of problems that technologists can, and will, encounter in everyday practice. Some of the questions are easy, some of them are not. In either case, the book is not only designed to test the reader's knowledge. It should also be used as tool to learn and understand nuclear medicine in preparation for passing nuclear medicine technology examinations. It is said that a picture is worth a thousand words. Our book includes more than 60 images, graphics, and diagrams. It is our goal for these illustrations to help the reader get to the bottom of the problem and come up with the right solution quicker.

The book is divided into seven chapters. We kick off the book with a chapter on test taking strategies. It is designed to equip you with practical tools and methods to successfully navigate through the multiple-choice exam. It was written by a recent graduate; the hands-on experience provides readers with valuable insider tips.

Chapters 2, 3, and 4 contain the test problems. Each sample test includes 220 multiple choice questions – chapters are organized in three levels of complexity, from the easiest to the most difficult. Generally, tagging questions as easy or difficult is a tricky matter, and highly subjective. Nevertheless, for learning purposes the proposed classification will be beneficial for readers. Each chapter is a separate entity with answers and optional short explanations included. This will work like building blocks, where the completion of the first test prepares the reader to progress to the second test, and so on.

Appendix A consists of the critical formulas, numbers, and normal range values for some of the quantitative nuclear medicine procedures. Some readers should commit these to memory – especially students preparing for licensee examinations – while others should at least be aware of where to locate them.

Appendix B offers a list of commonly used abbreviations and symbols that are encountered in daily nuclear medicine practice, and beyond. The list may either appear too short or too long; some readers may find the included terms unnecessary while other readers may not find the abbreviation they are looking for. One size never fits all, and thus it was a subjective choice in making the list – our selection is not comprehensive, but we think it is practical for review purposes. Use it to your advantage. There is enough space between the lines, and in the margins, to add or modify according to your own preference. Understanding the acronyms will pay off in the long run; simply being able to decode it, will be short-lived. Therefore, a thorough review of the abbreviations before the examinations can be very helpful, and highly suggested.

Appendix C is composed of Web site addresses that offer priceless and free information on many topics related to the nuclear medicine field. Our hope is that readers will explore them for more specific information.

The presented collection of problems closely mirrors the exam content as provided by NMTCB and ARRT. The questions cover radiation safety, radionuclides, and instrumentation to name a few. The reader should never be discouraged when the type of "never heard of" or "it is over my head" problem is encountered. We advise students to go through these questions carefully, and answer diligently – you will be surprised how much you already know and how much you still can learn. Both factors serve as great motivators. Learning should be fun, entertaining, and contagious. Nuclear medicine is a challenging and rapidly evolving field of medicine and the only way to keep pace with its development is through continuous learning. Make it fun, and make it a habit – this is the kind of addiction you can afford. You can read, you can study, you can investigate, and you can challenge yourself and others. Best of all you can exceed … your own expectations. The choice is yours.

IL, USA   Andrzej Moniuszko, MD, CNMT, ARRT(N), NCT, PET
                                                            Dharmesh Patel, CNMT, ARRT(N)

Acknowledgments

It is beyond the scope of words to express our appreciation to Dr. Adrian Kesala, Medical Director of Nuclear Medicine, Resurrection Medical Center, Chicago, for the opportunity of knowledge and his enthusiasm, suggestions, inspiration, and encouragement to write this book.

We want to thank Professor Joanne Metler, Coordinator of Nuclear Medicine Technology Program, College of DuPage, for her patience in reviewing our manuscript. Her dedication, helpful criticism, and detail-oriented effort deserve nothing but our sincere appreciation. Thank you for being with us through every chapter of our book.

We would also like to thank Mrs. Sabina Moniuszko for her devotion and intractable eagerness when preparing diagrams and drawings we used in throughout the book, and Mr. George Chang, PACS Coordinator, Resurrection Medical Center, Chicago for his priceless help in preparing clinical images.

Many thanks to our coworkers from the Nuclear Medicine Department at Resurrection Medical Center in Chicago for their assistance and for providing an environment that allowed us to write this guide.

Contents

Chapter 1
Tackling the Multiple-Choice Test

Marta L. Moniuszko

The Nuclear Medicine Technology exam is administered by two institutions: The American Registry of Radiologic Technologists (ARRT) and Nuclear Medicine Technology Certification Board (NMTCB). Once you choose either ARRT or NMTCB, the first step you should take is to visit their respective Web sites, and familiarize yourself with the test information provided that is specific to each. Think about a candy store. You can expect to buy sweets there, but the assortment, presentation, and the price will be different for each vendor. Make the effort to know the intimate details of ARRT's or NMTCB's exams. On the more "healthy" note, regardless of which one you choose to take your test with you will be taking a standard multiple-choice test administered on a computer. Multiple choice is the most common test format for standardized test, and it helps to understand the basic setup of this type of a test before tackling it.

A multiple-choice test is composed of three elements: stem, options, and distractors. The stem is the basic problem, and it may be either a question or an incomplete statement. Options are the list of responses available (NMTCB exam version has a five item list). The list contains one correct answer, and the remaining ones act as the distractors. The distractors are designed to appear as a plausible answer. You, as the test taker, must choose the best answers from the list of alternatives. Now, multiple-choice questions are, in fact, objective questions; they are based on information without the ambiguity of test taker's opinion or interpretation. This, coupled with the known and structured test format, allows the candidate to approach the test strategically.

Let us discuss the different methods and strategies for taking the multiple-choice test.

- Cover the list of responses with your hand, read the stem carefully, and actually try to answer the question before looking at the possible choices. By doing so, you will not be negatively influenced or confused by the available choices. Pick the response which best matches your initial answer.

M.L. Moniuszko (✉)
Systems Analyst, Aon Hewitt, Lincolnshire, IL, USA

A. Moniuszko and D. Patel, *Nuclear Medicine Technology Study Guide: A Technologist's Review for Passing Board Exams*, DOI 10.1007/978-1-4419-9362-5_1, © Springer Science+Business Media, LLC 2011

- Read the stem thoroughly (you can write down the important words), determine what is being asked, and then read all the answers carefully. Compare each choice to what you think is the correct answer, eliminate the obviously incorrect answers, and choose your answer from the remaining options.
- Another useful approach is to read the stem together with each of the options, one by one. Treat each combination as if it was a True/False question. If the combined statement is false, you can eliminate that option; if it appears to be correct mark it as a possible answer. Repeat this for all alternatives.
- For questions that are more complicated or difficult, try to simplify the stem, and summarize or rephrase the answers. In this way, both the stem and the options will be clearer, and make more sense to you, making the question more manageable.
- If none of the choices available to you match your predetermined answer, you can use one the following techniques to narrow down to the probable answer:

  - Usually, the positive answer or the longer/st response with most information is more likely to be the correct.
  - Responses containing phrases such as "All of the Above" or "None of the Above" are also more likely to be true. However, you must be careful. Do read all of the preceding responses and ensure all of them apply.
  - Be cautious of trap words such as "never," "every," "always," "only," and "completely." Read the alternatives containing these words very thoroughly. Keep in mind that options with absolute phrases suggest that the statement is always true, which is rarely correct.
  - On the other hand, words such as "may," "generally," "some," "usually," and "often" are clues that the answer might be correct.
  - Eliminate answers that are otherwise true but do not apply to the stem. In other words, if the option is only partially true or incorrect as it relates to the stem, reject it.
  - If two answers have similar one or two words or words that sound or look similar, choose one of the two.

- It is a good and advised practice to first answer the questions you are comfortable with, and not to get distracted if you cannot answer a question. Instead, tag each appropriately, and then to go back and reattempt to find the answers. Remember, the entire test is full of hints, and information contained in one part may help you in another.
- Keep in mind, usually your first choice is the correct one. Unless you determine based on information further along in the test or you are certain you misread the stem or the alternatives, you should not change your answer.
- If all of the above fails, guess, but do not guess until you have eliminated all of the definitely incorrect options. There is no penalty for incorrect answers.

In general, as it applies, you are not able to skip a question (leave it unanswered), but you may mark it, and come back to it later. You are also allowed to review your choices and change any answer before submitting the test. Each test administrator offers a brief test tutorial before the examination with sample questions. These are designed to help you familiarize yourself with the test process and the format of the questions.

Reading this section should arm you with a good selection of strategies to help you make your way through the multiple-choice test. Simultaneously, you are probably beginning to feel a slight hint of anxiety. The nervousness is likely to increase as you near your test exam date and will peak during the actual examination. It is just as equally important, therefore, to look into the arsenal of anxiety-fighting tools.

Tackling Test Anxiety

Preparation, both mental and physical, is said to be the number one killer of text anxiety. We will first explore this weapon.

There is a myriad of literature on the subject of studying methods. Having gotten as far as you have in your life, I trust you must have developed a good study technique that carried you this far. But for those who have been out of the study realm, let us review some of the basics of good study habits.

First of all, you must develop a study strategy. Depending on numerous factors, such as available time, time length before the exam, mental agility, and subject familiarity, the study plan will be different. Be realistic; you know what works for you and with your schedule, build the strategy accordingly. But remember, as Dwight D. Eisenhower once said in reference to preparation for a battle, "Plans are worthless, but planning is indispensable." Make plans and adjust them as your personal circumstances change. The most important thing is to continuously manage your study time and not to procrastinate. The study guide you hold in your hand is designed to help you navigate through the preparation. In a situation when you will find yourself lost in the piles of supplemental books, index cards, post-it notes or tape recorders, here are few study tips to get you back on track.

- Approach studying with positive attitude, and at the same time, eliminate any negative thoughts related to yourself or the actual studying.
- Arrange, or rearrange, your schedule to minimize any outside distractions. You should have a designated study area, preferably in a secluded, quite, and well-lighted place.
- Determine the part of the material you are going to study and for how long. Have everything ready and within reach, remove everything that is not related to the particular section. Stick to the plan.
- If you catch yourself day dreaming, or loosing concentration, switch to a different study area or subject.
- Take breaks. You can stretch, take a brisk walk, or eat a snack. Stop when you are feeling tired or are simply no longer productive.

This will take care of preparing mentally for the exam and reducing some of the anxiety that is uprooted from simply not being prepared. Just as importantly, you have to be physically ready. In general, the stronger the body is, the stronger the mind. Exercise throughout the entire study phase, but especially days before the examination. It will significantly reduce your stress level and improve brain function. Get a good night's sleep the night before the exam, and eat a nourishing breakfast. Your brain cannot operate without glucose and you will run out of energy without sufficient food in your body. Dress comfortably, preferably in layers so you are able to adjust your attire to the temperature inside the testing center. Prepare everything you need for the test the day ahead, and leave yourself ample time to arrive at the destination. Being mentally and physically prepared is bound to eliminate the majority of the test-related anxiety. There is, however, a small percentage of anxiety that will always be present in a high stakes environment. Accept it, it will actually help you stay alert and sharpen your mental reflexes.

On the day of the examination, it is critical to remain relaxed and release any mental or physical anxiety. To do so, arrive early to the test site, and do not study or review the material after your arrival. Rather, take a moment to yourself to perform couple of slow-breathing exercises, simultaneously visualize yourself at a peaceful place. This will allow you to stay calm and relaxed. During the examination, the outmost important thing is for you to concentrate on the question directly before. Do not fall into the trap of thinking about the question you just answered or the questions that follow. Your goal is to answer that question correctly. That is all that matters. The best tennis players win because they never let the ball out of their eye sight. Follow their winning practices. After the examination is completed, reflect back on your accomplishment and reward yourself!

Thomas A. Edison once said: "Many of life's failures are people who did not realize how close they were to success when they gave up." If he did give up, we might still be sitting in the dark. Don't. Good luck!

Suggested Readings

Gloe D. Study habits and test-taking tips. Dermatol Nurs. 1999;11:493–9.

Blackcy R. So many choices, so little time: strategies for understanding and taking multiple-choice exams in history. Hist Teach. 2009;43(1):53–66.

Kubistant T. Test performance: the neglected skill. Education. 2001;102(1):53–5.

Test taking power strategies. Learning Express, New York, NY, 2007.

Study Guides and Strategis. Overcoming test anxiety. http://www.studygs.net/tstprp8.htm. Accessed 12 Sept 2010.

Taking Multiple Choice Exams. http://www.uwec.edu/geography/Ivogeler/multiple.htm. Accessed 20 Sept 2010.

Chapter 2
Practice Test #1: Difficulty Level – Easy*

Questions

1. The venous blood returning via the superior vena cava (SVC) and inferior vena cava (IVC) enters the heart at the:
   - (A) Left atrium (LA)
   - (B) Right atrium (RA)
   - (C) Left ventricle (LV)
   - (D) Right ventricle (RV)

2. The mechanism by which the epithelial cells of the thyroid concentrate iodide is termed:
   - (A) Diffusion
   - (B) Hormonogenesis
   - (C) Active transport
   - (D) Absorption

3. Flood field nonuniformity in reconstructed SPECT images can result in:
   - (A) Star artifacts
   - (B) Ring artifacts
   - (C) Hot spot artifacts
   - (D) Cold spot artifacts

---

*Answers to Test #1 begin on page 54.

A. Moniuszko and D. Patel, *Nuclear Medicine Technology Study Guide: A Technologist's Review for Passing Board Exams*, DOI 10.1007/978-1-4419-9362-5_2, © Springer Science+Business Media, LLC 2011

4. Tc-99m Sulfur colloid can be used in all of the following types of imaging EXCEPT:
   (A) Bone marrow imaging
   (B) Gastrointestinal bleeding imaging
   (C) Liver imaging
   (D) Brain imaging

5. Figure 2.1 presents the diagrams of end-systolic (dashed line) and end-diastolic (solid line) shape of left ventricle cineangiogram. The drawing "a" represents normal left ventricle wall motion. What left ventricle abnormality corresponds to the drawing "b"?
   (A) Hypokinetic left ventricle
   (B) Hyperkinetic left ventricle
   (C) Akinetic left ventricle
   (D) Dyskinetic left ventricle

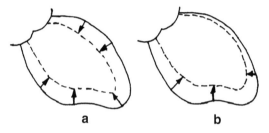

a   b

Fig. 2.1 End-systolic (dashed line) and end-diastolic (solid line) shape of left ventricle cineangiogram (*Illustration by Sabina Moniuszko*)

6. Popular radiation safety acronym ALARA stands for:
   (A) As Low as Radiologist Approve
   (B) As Low as Radiation Accepted
   (C) As Low as Reasonably Achievable
   (D) As Low as Reasonably Accepted

7. Technetium-99m is used in the majority of all standard nuclear medicine studies because Tc-99m:
   (A) Has a long half-life
   (B) Produces alpha and beta particles
   (C) Causes septal penetration
   (D) Provides good tissue penetration

8. A dose calibrator is used to assay the amount of a radioactivity in a sample before it is administered to a patient. All radiation leaving the source placed in the dose calibrator is detected EXCEPT radiation directed toward:
   (A) The bottom of the chamber
   (B) The hole at the top
   (C) The bottom half of the chamber
   (D) The upper part of the chamber

9. If expected value of the long-lived source is 120 μCi and actual reading obtained from dose calibrator is 122 μCi, what is the percentage error of that reading?
   (A) −2
   (B) −1.7
   (C) 1.7
   (D) 2.0

10. The size of the colloid particles is important in imaging the reticuloendothelial system. Particles smaller than 20 nm tend to accumulate in:
    (A) The bone marrow
    (B) The liver
    (C) The spleen
    (D) The lymph nodes

11. The cardiac measurement defined as the blood volume pumped out by the ventricle over 1 min time period is called the:
    (A) Ejection fraction
    (B) Stroke volume
    (C) Cardiac output
    (D) Systolic

12. Esophageal transit scintigraphy is fast, noninvasive, and easy to perform diagnostic procedure but its widespread use is limited because of:
    (A) High radiation exposure
    (B) Lack of standardization
    (C) Labeling difficulties
    (D) Food allergies

13. The daily quality control for dose calibrator includes a constancy check typically performed with small amounts of Cobalt-57 or Cesium-137. Cs-137 has a half-life of 30 years and produces:
    (A) 133 keV gamma ray
    (B) 388 keV gamma ray
    (C) 637 keV gamma ray
    (D) 662 keV gamma ray

14. Scintigraphy is the gold standard measurement of gastric emptying for diagnosis of gastroparesis. All the following symptoms are common among patients with gastric dysmotility disorders EXCEPT:
    (A) Nausea and vomiting
    (B) Early satiety
    (C) Abdominal bloating
    (D) Tachycardia

15. Figure 2.2 presents the schematic drawing of normal heart conduction system. The label "a" represents:
    (A) The left bundle branch
    (B) The right bundle branch
    (C) The sinoatrial node
    (D) The atrioventricular node

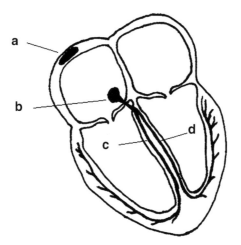

Fig. 2.2 Normal heart conduction system (*Illustration by Sabina Moniuszko*)

16. The Nuclear Regulatory Commission (NRC) has provided complete guidelines for retention of all records generated in a nuclear medicine department. Which of the following documentation should be kept indefinitely?
    (A) Misadministrations records
    (B) Patient dosage records
    (C) Personnel monitoring records
    (D) Sealed-source inventory records

17. The radionuclides emitting β particles should be stored in containers of low Z material to prevent:
    (A) Compton scatter
    (B) Bremsstrahlung radiation
    (C) Back injuries
    (D) Extra expenditures

18. The mathematical process of applying a negative value to both sides of the density histogram of each ray sum is called convolution filtering and is used in reconstruction method called:
    (A) Filtered backprojection
    (B) Iterative reconstruction
    (C) Ordered subset expectation maximization
    (D) Fourier transformation

19. 580 Microcuries (μCi) is equal to:
    (A) 58 curies (Ci)
    (B) 0.580 curie (Ci)
    (C) 0.00058 curie (Ci)
    (D) 0.000058 curie (Ci)

20. Fever of unknown origin (FUO) can be caused by all of the following disorders/factors EXCEPT:
    (A) Stress
    (B) Infection
    (C) Neoplasm
    (D) Drugs

21. When approaching unresponsive victim her/his occasional gasps the rescuer should:
    (A) Give rescue breath
    (B) Treat the victim gasps as effective breaths
    (C) Call 911
    (D) Wait till breathing become more regular

22. Tc-99m methylene diphosphonate (MDP) is the most widely used bone imaging agent. Uptake of the tracer depends on all of the following EXCEPT:
    (A) Local blood flow
    (B) Osteoblastic activity
    (C) Extraction efficiency
    (D) Liver function

23. The extrinsic flood image evaluates the uniformity of:
    (A) Detector only
    (B) Detector and collimator
    (C) Collimator only
    (D) Neither detector nor collimator

24. All of the following structures can be seen on a normal bone scan of the thorax
    region EXCEPT:
    (A) Sternoclavicular joint
    (B) Body of scapulae
    (C) Manubrium sternum
    (D) Sternal foramina

25. Presented images (Fig. 2.3) are example of what type of nuclear medicine
    acquisition?
    (A) Dynamic study
    (B) Static imaging
    (C) Dual point imaging
    (D) Flow study

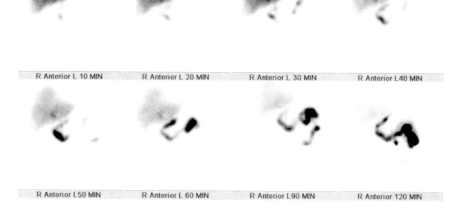

Fig. 2.3 Nuclear medicine acquisition

26. All of the following are recommended means of reducing radiation exposure
    EXCEPT:
    (A) Use of remote handling devices
    (B) Applying shielding
    (C) Wearing film badge
    (D) Limitation of time

27. One of two or more different nuclides having the same mass number is called:
    (A) Isomer
    (B) Isotope
    (C) Isobar
    (D) Isotone

28. All of the following quality control (QC) tests are performed in nuclear medi-
    cine department to assess the reproducibility of radiation counter EXCEPT:
    (A) The relative error
    (B) The chi-squared test
    (C) The reliability factor
    (D) The constancy test

29. A radioactive source produces exposure of 30 millirem per hour (mR/h) at
    2-m distance. If the distance is increased to 5-m what is the new exposure rate?
    (A) 4.8 mR/h
    (B) 5.1 mR/h
    (C) 5.6 mR/h
    (D) 6.1 mR/h

30. Excessive free pertechnetate in Tc-99m methylene diphosphonate (MDP)
    preparation will result in increased tracer accumulation in the:
    (A) Thyroid and stomach
    (B) Thyroid and kidney
    (C) Thyroid and bowel
    (D) Thyroid and liver

31. All of the following symptoms can be related to thyroid dysfunction
    EXCEPT:
    (A) Weight loss
    (B) Weight gain
    (C) Back pain
    (D) Irregular menstrual cycles

32. Extravasation of the tracer at the site of injection when performing bone scin-
    tigraphy may result in visualization of the:
    (A) Thyroid
    (B) Stomach
    (C) Kidney(s)
    (D) Lymph node(s)

33. The basic unit commonly used for expressing amounts of binary-coded information is called:
    (A) The bit
    (B) The byte
    (C) The word
    (D) The sequence

34. Tc-99m-labeled erythrocytes and Tc-99m sulfur colloid are two commonly used techniques to detect:
    (A) Active bleeding
    (B) Hemangioma
    (C) Melena
    (D) Hematemesis

35. Presented images (Fig. 2.4) are example of what type of nuclear medicine acquisition?
    (A) Dynamic study
    (B) Static imaging
    (C) Dual point imaging
    (D) SPECT study

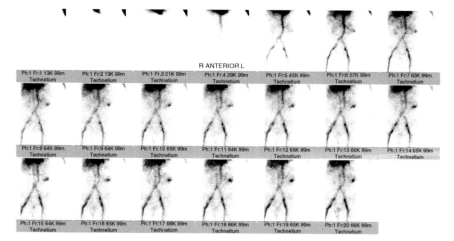

Fig. 2.4 Nuclear medicine acquisition

36. The diagnostic and therapeutic uses of radiopharmaceuticals are dependent on the accumulation of the material in the "organ of interest." According to the Nuclear Regulatory Commission (NRC) definition, the part of the body that is most susceptible to radiation damage under the specific conditions under consideration is called:

    (A) The critical organ
    (B) The paired organ
    (C) The target organ
    (D) The internal organ

37. A specific radiolabeled molecule that resembles the in vivo behavior of a natural molecule and can be used to provide information about a specific biological process is called:

    (A) Isotope
    (B) Radiotracer
    (C) Ligand
    (D) Pharmaceutical

38. The dose calibrator's ability to measure accurately a range of low-activity doses to high-activity doses is called:

    (A) Accuracy
    (B) Constancy
    (C) Geometry
    (D) Linearity

39. If cardiac net end-diastolic counts are 65,450 and net end-systolic counts are 31,219, what is the left ventricle ejection fraction?

    (A) 74%
    (B) 52%
    (C) 40%
    (D) 35%

40. All of the following findings on the gastrointestinal bleeding scintigraphy have the potential to reduce the specificity of the test EXCEPT:

    (A) Horse-shoe kidney
    (B) Dilated abdominal aorta
    (C) Hepatic hemangioma
    (D) Foreign body

41. Soaps are detergent-based products and are available in various forms includ-
    ing bar soap, tissue, leaflet, and liquid preparations. Which of the following
    statements regarding soaps and handwashing is false?
    (A) Handwashing with plain soap can result in increases in bacterial counts on
        the skin
    (B) Plain soaps have minimal antimicrobial activity
    (C) In many studies, handwashing with plain soap failed to remove pathogens
        from the hands of hospital personnel
    (D) Plain soaps cannot be contaminated

42. Cinegraphic loop viewing of dynamic images of the gastrointestinal bleeding
    scintigraphy:
    (A) Help to localize the site of bleeding
    (B) Eliminate the need of angiography
    (C) Have prognostic value
    (D) Is time consuming

43. Calibration, sensitivity/constancy, efficiency, chi-square, and energy resolution
    are quality control procedures performed to ensure proper operation of the:
    (A) Survey meter
    (B) Dose calibrator
    (C) Gamma-camera
    (D) Well counter and uptake probe

44. Which of the following gastrointestinal structures is more variable in location
    and more prone to overlap with vascular structures?
    (A) Stomach
    (B) Small bowel
    (C) Colon
    (D) Rectum

45. Images presented in Fig. 2.5 were acquired during routine bone scintigraphy
    and they should be labeled:
    (A) (a) and (b) – posterior views
    (B) (a) – anterior and (b) – posterior view
    (C) (a) – posterior and (b) – anterior view
    (D) (a) and (b) – anterior views

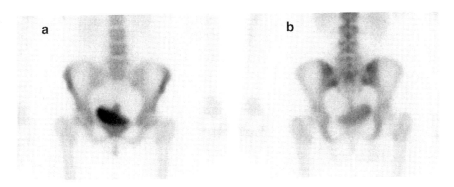

Fig. 2.5 Bone scintigraphy

46. Measurement of radioactive materials present inside a person's body through analysis of the person's blood, urine, feces, or sweat is called:

    (A) Radioconcentration
    (B) Biodosimetry
    (C) Biodistribution
    (D) Bioassay

47. The fraction of total radioactivity present in the form of desired radiopharmaceutical is called:

    (A) Formulation strength
    (B) Radionuclide purity
    (C) Integrity of a formulation
    (D) Radiochemical purity

48. The photons, after passing through the collimator interact with the sodium iodide crystal detector and produce pulses of light that are detected by the:

    (A) Scintillating solution
    (B) Photomultiplier tubes
    (C) Pulse height analyzer
    (D) Amplifier

49. Half-value layer of Tc-99m is 0.27 mm. If an unshielded vial of Tc-99m producing the exposure rate of 225 mR/h is placed in a storage area with lead shield that is 0.8 mm thick, what would be the new exposure rate?

    (A) 75 mR/h
    (B) 45 mR/h
    (C) 28 mR/h
    (D) 18 mR/h

50. Radiolabeled colloidal or macroaggregate particles should have a proper size range for a specific organ uptake. Tc-99m macroaggregated albumin (MAA) particles size from 10 to 100 μm:
    (A) Block the capillaries in lungs
    (B) Are taken up by the cells of reticuloendothelial system (RES) in liver and spleen
    (C) Are taken up by the cells of reticuloendothelial system (RES) in bone marrow
    (D) Block the arterioles in lungs

51. The mixture of thick semifluid mass of partly digested food and secretions that is passed from the stomach to the duodenum is called:
    (A) Bolus
    (B) Chyme
    (C) Ganglion
    (D) Chyle

52. The raw myocardial perfusion projection images are routinely evaluated for all of the following purposes EXCEPT:
    (A) Attenuation artifacts
    (B) Motion artifacts
    (C) Wall motion analysis
    (D) Noncardiac pathology

53. High-count floods performed on gamma-cameras are applied to:
    (A) Static images
    (B) Static and dynamic images only
    (C) SPECT images
    (D) Static, dynamic, and SPECT images

54. In-111 and Tc-99m-labeled white blood cells (WBC) accumulation have been observed in all of the following conditions/sites EXCEPT:
    (A) Gastrointestinal bleeding
    (B) Debridement sites
    (C) Vascular access lines
    (D) Focal seizures

55. Images presented in Fig. 2.6 were acquired during gated equilibrium radionuclide ventriculography and displayed as a splash view of myocardial cycle. How many frames per R–R interval were acquired during the acquisition?
    (A) 4
    (B) 8
    (C) 16
    (D) 32

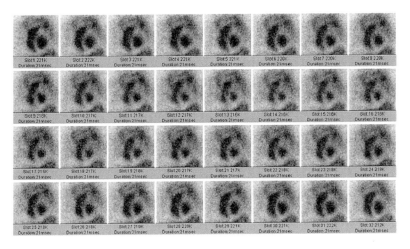

Fig. 2.6 Splash view of myocardial cycle

56. The relationship that states that electromagnetic radiation intensity is inversely proportional to the square of the distance from a point source is called:

    (A) Inverse square principle
    (B) Inverse square rule
    (C) Inverse square law
    (D) Inverse square protection

57. Tl-201 as thallous chloride at neutral pH with respect to biochemistry and physiology is considered to behave similarly to:

    (A) Sodium
    (B) Calcium
    (C) Potassium
    (D) Gallium

58. The Pulmonex Xenon System is commonly used to perform lung ventilation studies. Which part of the xenon trap system is responsible for trapping the radioactivity?

    (A) The Drierite
    (B) The mask
    (C) The charcoal filter
    (D) Soda lime crystals

59. What is the effective half-life of an isotope, that has a physical half-life of 18 h and a biological half-life of 10 h?

    (A) 2.5 h
    (B) 6.4 h
    (C) 7.5 h
    (D) 9.2 h

60. Tc-99m-labeled leukocytes and Tc-99m sulfur colloid accumulate in the reticuloendothelial cells of the bone marrow. The distribution of marrow activity is similar in all of the following conditions with the exception of:
    (A) Paget's disease
    (B) Bone fracture
    (C) Osteomyelitis
    (D) Shin splint

61. If the medication is injected at a 45-degree angle using a 5/8 in. needle with a 25 gauge, the injection is called:
    (A) Subcutaneous injection
    (B) Intramuscular injection
    (C) Intradermal injection
    (D) Intravenous injection

62. Tc-99m-labeled red blood cells (Tc-99m RBC's) and Tc-99m-labeled sulfur (Tc-99m SC) can be used for the detection of gastrointestinal bleeding. Which of the following statements correctly describe their properties?
    (A) Tc-99m RBC is rapidly cleared from intravascular space
    (B) Tc-99m RBC do not contribute to observed background activity
    (C) Tc-99m SC is rapidly cleared from intravascular space
    (D) Tc-99m SC use is limited for the detection of gastric bleeding only

63. The Positron emission tomography (PET) blank scan should be acquired and checked:
    (A) Daily
    (B) Weekly
    (C) Monthly
    (D) Annually

64. In the radionuclide localization of acute gastrointestinal bleeding, two radiopharmaceuticals – Tc-99m-labeled red blood cells and Tc-99m-labeled sulfur colloid – are commonly used. Tc-99m RBCs have a stable persistence within the blood pool. On the contrary, Tc-99m SC is rapidly cleared from intravascular space with a HALF-TIME of approximately:
    (A) 30–40 min
    (B) 20–30 min
    (C) 2–3 min
    (D) 3–10 s

65. Images presented in Fig. 2.7 were acquired during routine whole body bone scintigraphy after intravenous 25.7 mCi of Tc-99m methylene diphosphonate (MDP) administration. Which of the following statements is most consistent with the finding from the scan?

(A) Normal scan
(B) Ribs fractures
(C) Bone metastasis
(D) Paget's disease

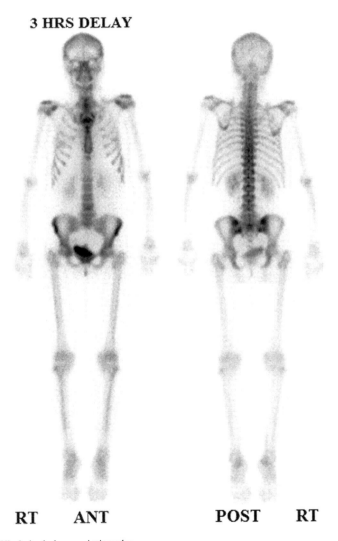

Fig. 2.7 Whole body bone scintigraphy

66. The increasing mean age of the US population and emerging new technologies will likely increase the demand for all of the following nuclear medicine procedures EXCEPT:
    (A) Tumor scans
    (B) Bone scans
    (C) Cardiac scans
    (D) Ventilation/perfusion scans

67. The major types of radiation listed by decreasing mass are:
    (A) γ, α, β
    (B) α, β, γ
    (C) α, γ, β
    (D) γ, β, α

68. The shield and the decay method are two different approaches to evaluate:
    (A) Effective dose measurement
    (B) γ-Camera linearity
    (C) Half-value layer thickness
    (D) Dose-calibrator linearity

69. If a study of 40 frames is acquired in BYTE mode on 128×128 matrix, what is the memory used if the acquisition is stored in WORD mode?
    (A) 327,680 words
    (B) 655,360 words
    (C) 655,360 bytes
    (D) 327,680 bytes

70. Sludge in the gallbladder is a common ultrasonographic finding in patients with chronic understimulation of the gallbladder. Sludge is:
    (A) Lithogenic bile
    (B) Acid chyme
    (C) Bile soap
    (D) Surfactant

71. Measurements used to assess the patient's condition are called the vital signs, and consist of the following vital parameters EXCEPT:
    (A) Blood pressure
    (B) Respiration rate
    (C) Temperature
    (D) Height and weight

72. False-positive cholescintigraphy can be minimized by a familiarity with its common causes. All of the following can elicit false-positive gallbladder scintigraphy results EXCEPT:

(A) Nonfasting
(B) Prolonged fasting
(C) Hepatocellular disease
(D) Dose extravasation

73. New imaging geometries using cadmium–zinc–telluride (CZT) detectors when compared with the parallel collimated Anger cameras:

(A) Have the same count sensitivities
(B) Have the same energy resolution
(C) Have the same spatial resolution
(D) Allow greatly reduced injected radioactivity

74. Relevant laboratory tests before performing bone scintigraphy, such as prostate-specific antigen (PSA) in patients with prostate cancer, frequently are performed. Which of the following laboratory blood tests can indicate bone pathology?

(A) Elevated BUN
(B) Elevated alkaline phosphatase
(C) Elevated aspartate aminotransferase
(D) Elevated troponin

75. Images presented in Fig. 2.8 acquired during routine bone scintigraphy after intravenous 24.1 mCi of Tc-99m methylene diphosphonate (MDP) administration. Which of the following statements is most consistent with the findings from the scan?

(A) Normal scan
(B) Rib fractures
(C) Bone metastases
(D) Paget's disease

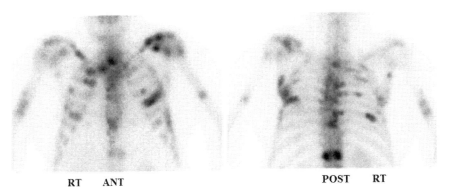

RT   ANT   **POST   RT**

Fig. 2.8 Bone scintigraphy

76. According to the American Society of Nuclear Cardiology (ASNC) recommendations, all of the following can result in reducing radiation exposure and obtaining high-quality diagnostic images EXCEPT:
    (A) Radiopharmaceutical selection
    (B) Individualized dose adjustment
    (C) Applying iterative reconstruction
    (D) Improving report turnaround time

77. The maximum permissible limit of Al^{+3} in Tc-99m eluate is set by:
    (A) U.S. Pharmacopeia
    (B) Nuclear Regulatory Commission (NRC)
    (C) Food and Drug Administration (FDA)
    (D) Society of Nuclear Medicine (SNM)

78. Leak testing on sealed sources, e.g., dose calibrator standards, spot markers, etc. must be performed at intervals not to exceed:
    (A) 1 week
    (B) 1 month
    (C) 6 months
    (D) 12 months

79. When performing a bone scan with Tc-99m methylene diphosphonate (MDP), the technologist sets the pulse height analyzer to 20% window. What is the acceptable energy range in this setting?
    (A) 126–154 keV
    (B) 112–168 keV
    (C) 120–160 keV
    (D) 130–150 keV

80. Abdominal pain during hepatobiliary scintigraphy with sincalide infusion:
    (A) Is predictive of the gallbladder disease
    (B) Is determined by the method of sincalide infusion
    (C) Is determined by the dose of radiopharmaceutical
    (D) Is predictive of the postcholecystectomy complications

81. All of the following organs belong to the urinary system EXCEPT:
    (A) The bladder
    (B) The urethra
    (C) The urethers
    (D) The uterus

82. The presence of a focal defect on rest images that was not seen on stress images, or the presence a focal defect on stress images that appears more severe on rest images is called:
    (A) Reverse redistribution
    (B) Viability image
    (C) Pseudo aneurysm
    (D) Cardiomyopathy

83. Every received package holding radioisotopes must be logged in properly. The incoming package logbook must include all of the following data EXCEPT:
    (A) Product name
    (B) Date
    (C) Driver's name
    (D) Received activity

84. The inferior wall of the left ventricle commonly demonstrates a decreased count density most likely caused by photons attenuation. All of the following can cause attenuation artifacts in the inferior wall of the left ventricle EXCEPT:
    (A) The left diaphragm
    (B) The right ventricle wall
    (C) The right ventricle blood pool
    (D) The right diaphragm

85. Display on the Fig. 2.9 presents reconstruction reoriented single photon emission computed tomography (SPECT MPI) data and created:
    (A) Short axis slices
    (B) Vertical long axis slices
    (C) Long axis slices
    (D) Horizontal long axis

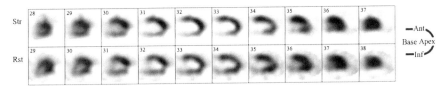

Fig. 2.9 Reconstruction reoriented SPECT MPI slices

86. Which of the following diagnostic examinations will deliver the smallest estimated dose to the fetus?
    (A) Abdomen CT
    (B) Pelvis X-ray
    (C) Interventional fluoroscopically guided procedures
    (D) Lung perfusion scan

87. The distance that the positron passes from its origin to the point of the annihilation is called:
    (A) Positron attenuation
    (B) Positron range
    (C) Travel range
    (D) Annihilation delay

88. Photomultiplier tube (PMT) consists of a photocathode and a series of dynodes in an evacuated glass enclosure. PMT converts:
    (A) The light photons into an electrical signal
    (B) An electrical signal into light
    (C) An electrical signal into heat
    (D) Heat into light

89. 850 milligrays (mGy) are equal to:
    (A) 0.850 rad
    (B) 85 rads
    (C) 85,000 rads
    (D) 8,500,000 rads

90. Attenuation artifacts of tomographic myocardial perfusion imaging may decrease the diagnostic accuracy of the technique, predominantly due to:
    (A) Increase in false negative
    (B) Increase in false positive
    (C) Increase in true negative
    (D) Increase in true positive

91. Kupffer cells of the liver are responsible for the radiopharmaceutical:
    (A) Extraction
    (B) Excretion
    (C) Phagocytosis
    (D) Breakdown

92. If the time between two successive R points is 1 s, a beat length acceptance window of 100% allows accumulation of data from cardiac beats:
    (A) Having a duration 1,000 ms
    (B) Having a duration 1–1,000 ms
    (C) Having a duration 500–1,500 ms
    (D) All duration beats will be accepted

93. Compton scatter from the patient overlaps into the energy levels located:
    (A) Around the energy peak
    (B) At low energy side of the energy window
    (C) At high energy side of the energy window
    (D) At all levels of energy window

94. A defect that is present on stress images, and not seen or present to the lesser degree on resting images is called:
    (A) Reversible defect
    (B) Reverse defect
    (C) Fixed defect
    (D) Transient defect

95. Figure 2.10 presents the schematic diagram of the hepatobiliary tract. What part of the hepatobiliary tree represents label "b"?
    (A) Sphincter of Oddi
    (B) Cystic duct
    (C) Common bile duct
    (D) Common hepatic duct

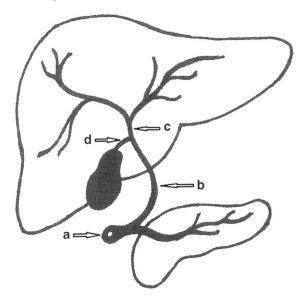

Fig. 2.10 Schematic diagram of hepatobiliary tract (*Illustration by Sabina Moniuszko*)

96. According to Nuclear Regulatory Commission-10 Code of Federal Regulations (NRC-10CFR) Part 20 Section 1201, a maximum permissible dose to extremities for radiation workers should not exceed:
    (A) 0.5 rem/year
    (B) 5 rem/year
    (C) 50 rem/year
    (D) 500 rem/year

97. The increasing distance between the origin of the positron and the location of the point of annihilation results in:
    (A) Attenuation artifact
    (B) Motion artifact
    (C) Decreased image resolution
    (D) Increased image resolution

98. The process of restricting the detection of emitted radiations to a given area of interest is called:
    (A) Attenuation
    (B) Collimation
    (C) Scattering
    (D) Pooling

99. How much activity will be remaining at 2:30 P.M. if the dose of Tc-99m methylene diphosphonate (MDP) is calibrated to contain 25 mCi at 12:00 P.M. on the same day?
    (A) 19.5 mCi
    (B) 18.7 mCi
    (C) 17.3.0 mCi
    (D) 15.7 mCi

100. Which of the following pharmacological stress agents is not approved by the US Food and Drug Administration (FDA) for stress testing in the USA?
    (A) Dobutamine
    (B) Adenosine triphosphate
    (C) Adenosine
    (D) Regadenoson

101. The brain consists of two hemispheres and each hemisphere has four lobes. Which of the following structures is NOT the brain's composition?
    (A) The frontal lobe
    (B) The lateral lobe
    (C) The parietal lobe
    (D) The temporal lobe

102. The methylxanthines competitively inhibit the adenosine receptors and can be a source of:
    (A) False-positive studies
    (B) False-negative studies
    (C) True-positive studies
    (D) True-negative studies

103. All of the following single photon emission computed tomography (SPECT) quality control procedures can be performed by the technologist EXCEPT:
    (A) Center of rotation (COR) calibration
    (B) Multiple head registration (MHR) validation
    (C) SPECT phantom
    (D) Uniformity correction matrix

104. A patient referred for Tc-99m mercaptoacetyltriglycine (MAG3) renal scintigraphy should:
    (A) Stay NPO (nothing per oral) for 6 h
    (B) Be well hydrated
    (C) Follow low carbohydrate diet
    (D) Avoid iodine containing medications

105. Figure 2.11 shows four different I-123 thyroid images where image (a) demonstrates a normal thyroid gland. The findings from image (b) are more consistent with the clinical diagnoses of:
    (A) Hypothyroidism
    (B) Grave's disease
    (C) Multinodular goiter
    (D) Autonomously hyperfunctioning thyroid nodule

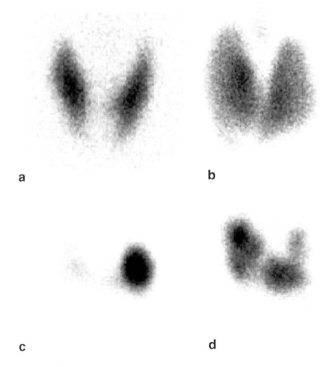

a   b

c   d

Fig. 2.11 I-123 thyroid scans

106. According to the criteria defining unrestricted areas and listed in Nuclear Regulatory Commission-10 Code of Federal Regulations (NRC-10CFR) Part 20 Section 1301, all licensees must perform procedures so that a dose in any unrestricted area does not exceed:

(A) 0.001 rem in any 1 h
(B) 0.002 rem in any 1 h
(C) 0.004 rem in any 1 h
(D) 0.005 rem in any 1 h

107. The product of the physical half-life and the decay constant is equal to:

(A) 0.5
(B) 0.693
(C) 0.693^2
(D) 1

108. The survey meter, also known as the Geiger-Mueller detector or Geiger counter, is a radiation detector filled with:

(A) Water
(B) Gas
(C) Lead
(D) Scintillation crystals

109. At the time of preparation, a macroaggregated albumin (MAA) kit contained 30.5 mCi of Tc-99m. How much activity will remain after 5 h and 30 min?

(A) 7.2 mCi
(B) 10.5 mCi
(C) 16.2 mCi
(D) 18.5 mCi

110. Technetium-labeled blood cells can be used in all of the following types of nuclear medicine scintigraphies EXCEPT:

(A) Hemangioma imaging
(B) Osteomyelitis imaging
(C) GI bleed scan
(D) Meckel's diverticulum scan

111. Obstruction of the passage of food through the mouth, pharynx, or the esophagus is called:

(A) Dyspepsia
(B) Dystrophia
(C) Dysphasia
(D) Dysphagia

112. Patient preparation for some of the nuclear medicine scintigraphies is essential. For all of the following NM imaging procedures, the patient has to remain NPO (nothing per oral) after midnight EXCEPT for the:
   (A) Gastroesophageal reflux study
   (B) Gastric empty scan
   (C) Liver–spleen scan
   (D) Hepatobiliary scan

113. The battery check, sealed source check, and calibration are three different quality control procedures performed to ensure proper operation of the:
   (A) Geiger-Mueller detector
   (B) Well counter
   (C) Thyroid probe
   (D) Glucose meter

114. The form of targeted radionuclide therapy that uses a monoclonal antibody to deliver localized radiation is called:
   (A) Radioimmunotherapy
   (B) Radiochemotherapy
   (C) Radiation therapy
   (D) Antibody therapy

115. Curves of cortical kidney activity are displayed in Fig. 2.12. Graph (a) presents a normal pattern with a prompt increase in activity and spontaneous washout. Curve of cortical kidney activity displayed on graph "B" is described as:
   (A) Dilated nonobstructed pattern
   (B) Blunted response pattern
   (C) Obstructed pattern
   (D) Golden pattern

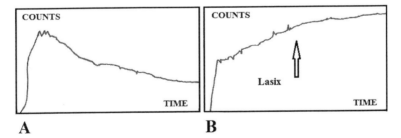

Fig. 2.12 Cortical kidney activity (*Illustration by Sabina Moniuszko*)

116. According to the Nuclear Regulatory Commission (NRC), an adult is defined as an individual:
    (A) 16 or more years of age
    (B) 18 or more years of age
    (C) 21 or more years of age
    (D) 23 or more years of age

117. An atom with an unstable nucleus is called a:
    (A) Radiochemical
    (B) Radionuclide
    (C) Radiopharmaceutical
    (D) Radio wave

118. The quality control procedure known as survey meter calibration is usually performed by:
    (A) The physicist
    (B) The technologist
    (C) The lead technologist
    (D) The radiation safety officer

119. If the net maximum counts of 67,670 and the net minimum counts of 25,659 are obtained from the region of interest (ROI) drawn over the gallbladder (GB) area, what is the calculated GB ejection fraction?
    (A) 22%
    (B) 32%
    (C) 52%
    (D) 62%

120. The general pretreatment requirements for adult qualifying for therapy with I-131 metaiodobenzylguanidine (MIBG) include the following EXCEPT:
    (A) A diagnostic MIBG scan or previous posttreatment I-131 MIBG scan
    (B) Reviewing potential interfering medications
    (C) Blocking thyroid uptake of free radioiodine
    (D) Performing pulmonary function tests

121. The most proximal part of the conduction system of the heart that exhibits the most automaticity is called:

   (A) The Purkinje fibers
   (B) The bundle of His
   (C) The sinus node
   (D) The atrioventricular node

122. All generic names for monoclonal antibodies end with the suffix "mab." Most frequently, the monoclonal antibodies are derived from:

   (A) Mouse
   (B) Fish
   (C) Rat
   (D) Human

123. To ensure the proper operation of the dose calibrator, all of the following quality control procedures must be performed on the unit EXCEPT:

   (A) Accuracy
   (B) Constancy
   (C) Battery check
   (D) Geometry

124. Human antimurine antibody (HAMA) is being produced when:

   (A) A murine immunoglobulin is injected into a mouse
   (B) A murine immunoglobulin is injected into a human
   (C) A humane immunoglobulin is injected into a mouse
   (D) A human immunoglobulin is injected into a human

125. Figure 2.13 displays the images obtained from 15-year-old-child 3-h post injection of Tc-99m methylene diphosphonate (MDP). What is the cause of the activity shown by the arrow?

   (A) Growth plate
   (B) Sports injury
   (C) Bad tagging
   (D) Osteoporosis

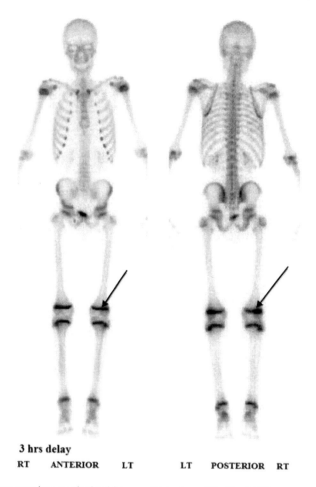

3 hrs delay

RT   ANTERIOR   LT   LT   POSTERIOR   RT

Fig. 2.13 Bone scan images obtained 3 hrs post injection of Tc 99m MDP

126. How often every organization is responsible for notifying each employee of his cumulative radiation dose?
    (A) Every week
    (B) Every month
    (C) Every 6 months
    (D) Once a year

127. When comparing the mass of an atom to the sum of the individual pieces of the atom, there will always be:
    (A) Less mass than expected
    (B) More mass than expected
    (C) No difference
    (D) Impossible to estimate

128. The quality control procedure performed on the dose calibrator with all the dose configurations used in the nuclear medicine department is called:
    (A) Accuracy
    (B) Linearity
    (C) Geometry
    (D) Constancy

129. If a 15 mCi of F-18 fluorodeoxyglucose (FDG) dose is needed for positron emission tomography (PET) scan at 1:00 P.M., how much activity should be prepared at 10 A.M.?
    (A) 4.8 mCi
    (B) 11 mCi
    (C) 21.2 mCi
    (D) 46.6 mCi

130. The hematologic toxicity of Y-90 Zevalin therapy is common. All of the following can be a sign of hematologic toxicity EXCEPT:
    (A) Fever
    (B) Bruising
    (C) Anemia
    (D) Arrhythmia

131. Pulmonary embolism (PE) usually is due to embolism of a thrombus (blood clot) The other possible embolic materials include all of the following EXCEPT:
    (A) Air
    (B) Globules of fat
    (C) Amniotic fluid
    (D) Saliva

132. The summed difference score (SDS) is derived as the difference between summed stress score (SSS) and summed rest score (SRS) and represents:
    (A) The reversibility of perfusion defects
    (B) The myocardial viability
    (C) The extend of the scar tissue
    (D) The left ventricle (LV) dilatation

133. The measure obtained by taking the counts per minute detected by the instrument and dividing them by the actual disintegrations per minute from the same source is called:
    (A) Counter accuracy
    (B) Counter efficiency
    (C) Counter reliability
    (D) Counter reproducibility

134. Many sulfur colloid kits contain ethylenediaminetetraacetic acid (EDTA), the chelating agent that binds the Al^{+3} ions and prevents:

    (A) The disintegration of the colloidal particles
    (B) The aggregation of the colloidal particles
    (C) The phagocytosis of the colloidal particles
    (D) The migration of the colloidal particles

135. The myocardial perfusion defect can be estimated by analyzing the stress-label (a) and the rest-label (b) images. The bull's eye polar plot images presented in Fig. 2.14a,b indicate the presence of:

    (A) Irreversible defect
    (B) Reversible defect
    (C) Scar tissue
    (D) Apical thinning

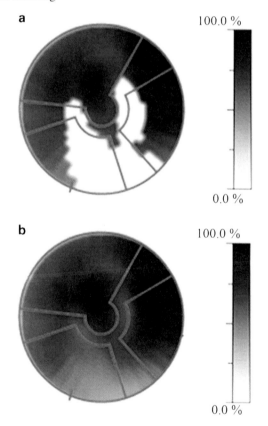

Fig. 2.14 Bull's-eye polar plot

136. Different level of radioactivities are handled in different areas of the nuclear medicine departments. Radioactivity in the range of microcurie levels are carried out in the section of NM department designated as:
    (A) Warm area
    (B) Hot area
    (C) Lukewarm area
    (D) Cold area

137. The minimum amount of energy needed to overcome the forces holding the atom together is called:
    (A) Holding energy
    (B) Binding energy
    (C) Kinetic energy
    (D) Thermal energy

138. The center of rotation (COR) of gamma-cameras is a key quality control procedure performed to assess capability of the nuclear medicine cameras to perform:
    (A) SPECT imaging
    (B) Planar imaging
    (C) Dual phase scanning
    (D) Dynamic scanning

139. A voiding cystogram is scheduled to be performed on a 5 year old child. Approximately how much saline (0.9% NaCl) should be infused into the patient's bladder during the procedure?
    (A) 330 ml
    (B) 270 ml
    (C) 240 ml
    (D) 210 ml

140. Regadenoson is an A_{2A} adenosine receptor agonist that dilates the coronary arteries. Lexiscan is supplied as a single use pre-filled syringe containing regadenoson:
    (A) 0.04 mg/ml
    (B) 0.08 mg/ml
    (C) 0.4 mg/ml
    (D) 0.8 mg/ml

141. The part of the large intestine, on the right side of the abdomen that extends from the cecum to the transverse colon, is called:
    (A) Sigmoid
    (B) Appendix
    (C) Ascending colon
    (D) Descending colon

142. Dose misadministration reports sent to the Nuclear Regulatory Commission (NRC) must include:
    (A) Patient name, age, gender
    (B) Patient name, age, gender diagnosis
    (C) Patient name, age, gender diagnosis, address
    (D) Information whether the patient or a relative was notified

143. The xenon trap machine and aerosol nebulizer are employed to perform lung ventilation studies. Which of the following quality control procedures are performed on the Xenon trap machine?
    (A) The Drierite freshness test
    (B) Soda lime crystals hygroscopic test
    (C) Charcoal filter consistency test
    (D) Xenon leak test

144. According to the "TechneScan MAG3" package, filtered air added to the reaction vial immediately following the addition of Tc-99m pertechnetate:
    (A) Oxidizes excess stannous ion
    (B) Reduces excess stannous ion
    (C) Evens out the pressure inside the reaction vial
    (D) Speeds up the formation of Tc-99m mertiatide

145. Figure 2.15 displays the images obtained during bone scintigraphy and shows arrow-excessive bladder activity, which can obscure underlying bone pathology. To obtain better quality images, technologist should:
    (A) Repeat images after voiding
    (B) Take lateral views
    (C) Use masking technique to exclude bladder from the image
    (D) Use lead plate to shield the bladder

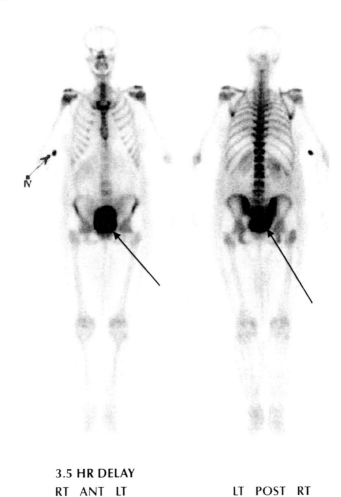

3.5 HR DELAY
RT ANT LT   **LT POST RT**

Fig. 2.15 Bone scintigraphy

146. Different levels of radioactivities are being handled in different areas of nuclear medicine departments. Radioactivities in the range of millicurie levels are carried out in the section of NM department designated as:
    (A) Warm area
    (B) Hot area
    (C) Lukewarm area
    (D) Cold area

147. Technetium-99m and technetium-99 are:
    (A) Isotones
    (B) Isobars
    (C) Isomers
    (D) Isotopes

148. When performing daily intrinsic floods, a point source of Tc-99m is placed five crystal dimensions away and centered over the detector. A point source should produce a measured counting rate not greater than:
    (A) 5,000 cps
    (B) 15,000 cps
    (C) 25,000 cps
    (D) 35,000 cps

149. A bone scan is scheduled to be performed with 25 mCi of Tc-99m methylene diphosphonate (MDP) at 12:30 P.M. How much Tc-99m MDP should be placed in the syringe at 8:00 A.M. on the same day?
    (A) 42 mCi
    (B) 37.4 mCi
    (C) 35 mCi
    (D) 33 mCi

150. Several materials for everyday use in the Nuclear medicine department have the expiration date listed on the package. Which of the following packages, with provided expiration dates, can be used safely on July 30, 2011?
    (A) Package with expiration date June 30, 2011
    (B) Package with expiration date May 30, 2011
    (C) Package with expiration date August 1, 2011
    (D) Package with expiration date July 1, 2011

151. The anatomical structure dividing the heart into two functionally separate and anatomically distinct units and separates left atrium and ventricle from the right atrium and ventricle is called:
    (A) Atrioventricular septum
    (B) Tricuspid valve
    (C) Bicuspid valve
    (D) Ventricular septum

152. Tc-99m and I-123 are the most commonly used agents for thyroid imaging. Thyroid imaging with technetium administration:
    (A) Cannot be performed with pinhole collimator
    (B) Requires 6 h delay evaluation
    (C) Doesn't require anti thyroid medications withholding
    (D) Does not evaluate true thyroid function

153. Co-57, Ge-68, and Ba-133 are sometimes called "mock" isotopes. Which of the following trios of isotopes do they imitate?

  (A) Tc-99m, I-131, Co-60
  (B) Tc-99m, F-18, I-131
  (C) Co-60, Xe-133, F-18
  (D) Xe-133, Ga-67, Sm-153

154. A lone "cold" nodule in an otherwise normal thyroid gland warrants:

  (A) Surgical removal
  (B) Fine needle aspiration biopsy
  (C) Radiation therapy
  (D) Chemotherapy

155. The images shown in Fig. 2.16 are acquired during routine bone scintigraphy. What is wrong with these pictures?

  (A) Wrong labels
  (B) Bad tag
  (C) Wrong radiopharmaceutical
  (D) There is nothing wrong with these images

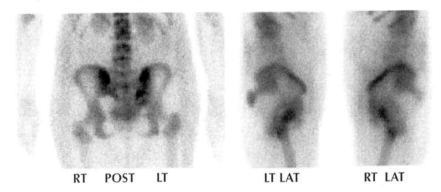

RT   POST   LT   LT LAT   RT LAT

Fig. 2.16 Bone scintigraphy

156. Oxygen radiosensitizes human cells to the damaging effects of radiation by:

  (A) Promoting cellular growth
  (B) Promoting cellular division
  (C) Promoting free radical production
  (D) Promoting cellular healing

157. In Compton scattering, the incoming photon scatters off an electron that is initially at rest. The electron gains energy and the scattered photon possess:
    (A) Lower energy, shorter wavelength
    (B) Lower energy, longer wavelength
    (C) Higher energy, shorter wavelength
    (D) Higher energy, longer wavelength

158. The gamma-camera is the most widely used imaging piece of equipment in nuclear medicine. The performance parameters of a routine gamma-camera quality control (QC) program include all of the following EXCEPT:
    (A) Spatial resolution
    (B) Peaking linearity
    (C) Energy resolution
    (D) Flood uniformity

159. A nuclear medicine department receives 375 mCi of Tc-99m in 4.5 ml bulk vial. If the macroaggregated albumin (MAA) kit is to be reconstituted with 30 mCi in 3 ml, how much saline should be added to the kit?
    (A) 1.64 ml
    (B) 2.64 ml
    (C) 3.0 ml
    (D) 3.6 ml

160. Esophageal activity can mimic ectopic thyroid tissue on a thyroid scan. To avoid misinterpretation:
    (A) Perform imaging with low energy, all purpose (LEAP) collimator
    (B) Repeat images after water ingestion
    (C) Repeat images with two markers
    (D) Repeat the scan in 2 weeks

161. The mediastinum is the space in the thoracic cavity behind the sternum and in between the two pleural sacs that contains all of the following anatomical structures EXCEPT:
    (A) Thyroid
    (B) Aorta
    (C) Trachea
    (D) Esophagus

162. To reduce radiation exposure to the patient undergoing radioactive iodine (RAI) treatment, all of the following recommendations will be helpful EXCEPT:
    (A) Patient should be well hydrated
    (B) Patient should urinate frequently
    (C) Patient laxatives
    (D) Patient should use antiperspirant medications

163. Spatial resolution and spatial linearity of a gamma-camera is assessed with a 4-quadrant bar phantom which consists of four sectors of lead bars and intervening plastic strips:
     (A) 1, 2, 3, and 4 mm in width
     (B) 2, 2.5, 3, and 4 mm in width
     (C) 2.5, 3, 4, and 4.5 mm in width
     (D) 3, 4, 5, and 6 mm in width

164. Ultrasound and radionuclide cholescintigraphy are commonly used in the process of evaluation of gallbladder disease. The main advantage of performing a hepatobiliary imino-diacetic acid (HIDA) scan over ultrasound is:
     (A) HIDA scan allows assessment of gallbladder function
     (B) HIDA scan takes less time to complete
     (C) HIDA scan allows gall stones measurements
     (D) HIDA scan can be performed during pregnancy

165. Figure 2.17 presents the images acquired during the first 4 h of the ventriculoperitoneal shunt patency study. What is the radiopharmaceutical most commonly used in this type of scintigraphy?
     (A) In-111 hexamethylpropyleneamine oxime
     (B) Tc-99m sulfur colloid
     (C) Tc-99m mercaptoacetyltriglycine
     (D) Tc-99m hydroxyiminodiacetic acid

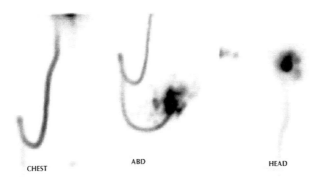

CHEST   ABD   HEAD

Fig. 2.17 Ventriculoperitoneal shunt patency study

166. Iodine-131 is considered to be the treatment of choice in many patients with Graves' disease. The most common side effect of radioactive iodine (RAI) treatment is:
     (A) Hyperthyroidism
     (B) Hypothyroidism
     (C) Thyroid carcinoma
     (D) Thyroiditis

167. Phosphorus-33, copper-67, iodine-131, and yttrium-90 are examples of:
    (A) Alpha-particle emitters
    (B) Beta-particle emitters
    (C) Alpha- and beta-particle emitters
    (D) Pure gamma emitters

168. Basic algorithms for reconstruction of tomographic images from projection figures include two analytic techniques known as:
    (A) Filtered backprojection and volume rendering techniques
    (B) Filtered backprojection and iterative techniques
    (C) Inverse Fourier transform and filtering techniques
    (D) Filtering and volume rendering techniques

169. If 300 μCi of I-123 is used for an adult dose, what is the pediatric dose according to Young's formula for a child who is 14-year old and weighs 65 lbs?
    (A) 250 μCi
    (B) 185 μCi
    (C) 173 μCi
    (D) 162 μCi

170. The period of time required for the concentration or amount of drug in the body to be reduced by 50% (percent) is known as:
    (A) Absorption time
    (B) Half-life
    (C) Therapeutic index
    (D) Potency

171. Slowed or stopped intravenous (IV) infusion, swelling, pain, and coldness around the needle site indicate:
    (A) Infiltration
    (B) Inflammation
    (C) Infection
    (D) Infraction

172. The most prevalent modes of myocardial perfusion imaging (MPI) tomographic acquisition are the "step-and-shoot" and "continuous technique." Small amount of blurring is present if the images are acquired by:
    (A) Step and shoot
    (B) Both methods
    (C) Continuous
    (D) Neither method

173. The reduction of image noise by reducing high-frequency information is called:
    (A) Fourier transform
    (B) Filtered backprojection
    (C) Filtering
    (D) Expectation maximization

174. Which of the following medications can be used as an adjunct to myocardial perfusion imaging (MPI) pharmacological stress testing?
    (A) Digoxin
    (B) Atropine
    (C) Coumadine
    (D) Aspirin

175. Images presented in Fig. 2.18 are acquired during routine liver–spleen scintigraphy. What is wrong with these images?
    (A) Wrong label
    (B) Bad tag
    (C) Wrong radiopharmaceutical
    (D) There is nothing wrong with these images

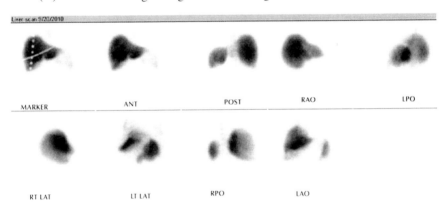

Fig. 2.18 Liver-spleen scintigraphy

176. All of the following are types of radioactive material licenses EXCEPT:
    (A) Specific
    (B) Broad
    (C) Wide
    (D) General

177. The nucleus is composed of two types of particles called:
    (A) Protons and electrons
    (B) Electrons and quarks
    (C) Neutrons and protons
    (D) Quarks and protons

178. References used to inform chemical users of the hazards associated with chemicals, and to advise users of the appropriate precautions, are known as:
    (A) Material Safety Data Sheet (MSDS)
    (B) Code of Federal Regulations (CFR)
    (C) Listing of United States Pharmacopeia (USP)
    (D) Regulations of United States Nuclear Regulatory Commission (U.S. NRC)

179. Xe-133, used during a ventilation/perfusion (VQ) scan has a physical half-life of 5.3 days and biological half-life is 0.37 min. What is the effective half-life of Xe-133?
    (A) 5.3 min
    (B) 3.7 min
    (C) 0.37 min
    (D) 5 s

180. All of the following radioisotopes have been approved in the USA for use in the treatment of bone metastases EXCEPT:
    (A) Strontium chloride Sr-89
    (B) Phosphorus P-32
    (C) Radium Ra-223
    (D) Samarium Sm-153

181. The liver is divided into four lobes based on surface features. Which of the following lobes is not the part of the liver?
    (A) The right lobe
    (B) The left lobe
    (C) The medium lobe
    (D) The caudate lobe

182. In which of the following causes of fever of unknown origin (FUO) diagnostic leukocyte scintigraphy may be especially valuable?
    (A) Systemic rheumatic disease
    (B) Infection
    (C) Neoplasm
    (D) Granulomatous disorder

183. The short axis cardiac tomogram is displayed with the orientation as if the viewer was observing the heart from the:
    (A) Base
    (B) Apex
    (C) Lateral wall
    (D) Inferior wall

184. All of the following can cause erroneous standardized uptake value (SUV) measurements EXCEPT:
    (A) Patient size
    (B) Injected dose
    (C) Plasma glucose level
    (D) Time of measurement

185. Presented below images were acquired 25 min after intravenous administration of 19.9 mCi of Tc-99m sestamibi. What type of nuclear medicine scintigraphy is displayed in Fig. 2.19?
    (A) Thyroid scan
    (B) Parathyroid scan
    (C) Salivary scan
    (D) Brain scan

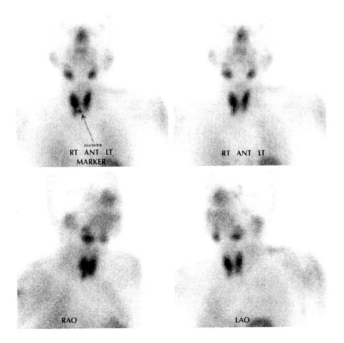

Fig. 2.19 Nuclear medicine scintigraphy obtained after intravenous administration of Tc-99m sestamibi

186. An individual responsible for the daily implementation of the radiation safety program in accordance with directives from the Radiation Safety Committee (RSC), license provisions, and regulatory requirements is named:
    (A) Senior Technologist
    (B) The Radiation Safety Officer (RSO)
    (C) Nuclear Medicine Physician
    (D) Chief Executive Officer (CEO)

187. Samarium-153 (Quadramet) is a therapeutic radiopharmaceutical used to treat:
    (A) Polycythemia vera
    (B) Medullary thyroid carcinoma
    (C) Dyspnea in lung Ca
    (D) Pain in bony metastases

188. Increasing the thickness of the scintillation detector will result in the detector:
    (A) Increased sensitivity and increased resolution
    (B) Increased sensitivity and decreased resolution
    (C) Decreased and increased resolution
    (D) Decreased and decreased resolution

189. If generator elute contains 635 mCi of Tc-99m, what is the maximum amount of Mo-99 allowed? (0.15 μCi Mo-99 per mCi Tc-99m)
    (A) 95.3 μCi
    (B) 64.2 μCi
    (C) 0.54 μCi
    (D) 0.15 μCi

190. Dual time-point imaging (DTPI) can improve accuracy of positron emission tomography (PET) imaging. DTPI technique is a specialized protocol in which:
    (A) Flow study is performed followed by static imaging
    (B) Two days delay imaging is performed
    (C) Dual-isotope technique is applied
    (D) Delay imaging is performed

191. Most patients with overt hyperthyroidism have an assemblage of symptoms which include all of the following EXCEPT:
    (A) Anxiety
    (B) Tremor
    (C) Weight loss
    (D) Decreased appetite

192. What is the predominant toxicity of radioisotopes used in the treatment of bone metastases?
    (A) Myelosuppression
    (B) Leukemia
    (C) Gastritis
    (D) Radiation pneumonitis

193. All of the following components of the scintillation camera are housed on the camera head EXCEPT:
    (A) Photomultiplier tubes
    (B) Touch pad
    (C) Display monitor
    (D) Amplifiers

194. Image representation of raw data obtained from projections of the object for image reconstruction is called:
    (A) Sinogram
    (B) Star artifact
    (C) Uniformity projections
    (D) Blank scan

195. Figure 2.20. A 57-years-old man with sudden onset of tachycardia and dyspnea and referred for lung scintigraphy. Displayed images were acquired after intravenous administration of 4.1 mCi of Tc-99m macroaggregated albumin (MAA). Which lung perfusion view demonstrates greatest cardiac shadow?
    (A) Posterior
    (B) Anterior
    (C) LPO
    (D) Left lateral

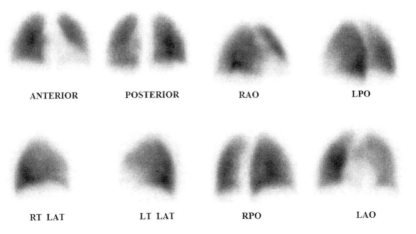

ANTERIOR   POSTERIOR   RAO   LPO

RT LAT   LT LAT   RPO   LAO

Fig. 2.20 Nuclear medicine lung perfusion scintigraphy

196. Dose equivalency is being measured in units called:
    (A) Curies
    (B) Rads
    (C) Rems
    (D) Becquerels

197. An alpha particle is identical to the nucleus of a helium atom. Alpha particles:
    (A) Are not charged
    (B) Travel unlimited distances
    (C) Are used for radionuclide therapy
    (D) Are smaller than beta particles

198. If the sample volume of a given activity is increased, the counting efficiency of the well counter will:
    (A) Decrease
    (B) Increase
    (C) Not change
    (D) Approach 0

199. Patient received 200 µCi of I-123 for thyroid uptake and scan. If the data shown below were obtained 6 h post administration of I-123, what is the percentage thyroid uptake at 6 h?

| 200 µCi I-123 capsules cts | 135,890 cpm | Background cts | 109 cpm |
| Thyroid cts | 45,534 cpm | Thigh cts | 2,109 cpm |

    (A) 25%
    (B) 28%
    (C) 32%
    (D) 68%

200. A significant enlargement in left ventricular (LV) size on the stress myocardial perfusion imaging (MPI) as compared to the rest images is called:
    (A) Transient Ischemic Dilation
    (B) Cardiomegaly
    (C) Hypertrophy
    (D) Hibernation

201. Blood pressure is expressed in units of:
    (A) Millimeters of mercury
    (B) Centimeters of mercury
    (C) Millimeters of blood
    (D) Centimeters of blood

202. In order to correctly calculate gallbladder ejection fraction, the GB must be:
    (A) Free of superimposition
    (B) Distended
    (C) Free of stones
    (D) Dyskinetic

203. Which of the following quality control procedures is NOT performed to ensure proper operation of the survey meter?
    (A) Battery check
    (B) Sealed source check
    (C) Accuracy
    (D) Calibration

204. If a patient has an irregular heart rate, the total number of cardiac cycles acquired for each projection will be the same if each projection is acquired for:
    (A) The same length of time
    (B) The same number of beats
    (C) The same number of counts
    (D) The same acceptance window

205. A 48-year-old woman with an abnormal treadmill stress test result, and a history of abdominal surgery, referred for a myocardial perfusion study. Figure 2.21 displays the resting raw projections of SPECT obtained after 3.2 mCi of Tl-201 administration. The images are consistent with the patient's surgical history of:
    (A) Splenectomy
    (B) Right nephrectomy
    (C) Left nephrectomy
    (D) Hysterectomy

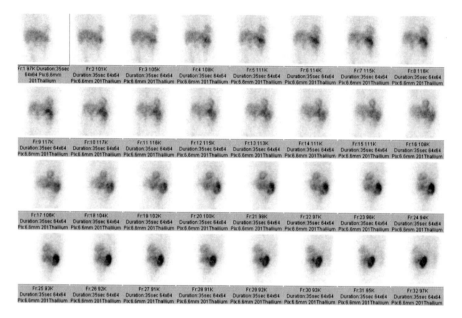

Fig. 2.21 Myocardial perfusion study-resting raw projections after Tl-201 administration

206. Which of the following patients undergoing diagnostic medical procedures are considered as a radioactive source?
    (A) Patient undergoing MRI study with gadolinium administration
    (B) Patient undergoing CT scan with iodine administration
    (C) Patient undergoing NM study with radiopharmaceutical administration
    (D) Patient undergoing X-ray study

207. In isomeric transition decay, the extra energy in the nucleus is released by the emission of:
    (A) X rays
    (B) Electrons
    (C) Gamma photons
    (D) Neutrons

208. When only image quality is considered, the best possible distance between the collimator and the patient's body for a gamma-camera equipped with HRES collimator is:
    (A) 10 cm
    (B) Half the collimator diameter
    (C) Contact
    (D) 1 in.

209. Large I-131 therapy dose stored in a nuclear medicine department produces an exposure of 80 mR/h. What thickness of lead is required to reduce the exposure rate to less than 1 mR/h? HVL for I-131 is 0.21 mm.

(A) 1.0 mm
(B) 1.5 mm
(C) 2.0 mm
(D) 2.1 mm

210. The primary route of excretion of Tc-99m hexakis 2-metoxy isobutyl isonitrile (Sestamibi) is:

(A) Skin
(B) Hepatobiliary tract
(C) Urinary tract
(D) Respiratory tract

211. The myocardium, in a typical fasting state, primarily uses as a substrate:

(A) Glucose
(B) Free fatty acids
(C) Proteins
(D) Aminoacids

212. "Single isotope dual phase technique" commonly applied in parathyroid imaging is based on the observation that:

(A) Tl-201 washes out more rapidly from the thyroid than from abnormal parathyroid
(B) Tl-201 washes out more rapidly from the abnormal parathyroid than from thyroid
(C) Tc-99m MIBI washes out more rapidly from the thyroid than from abnormal parathyroid
(D) Tc-99m MIBI washes out more rapidly from the abnormal parathyroid than from thyroid

213. The usefulness of F-18 FDG PET in infection imaging is based on the fact that granulocytes and macrophages in infectious foci:

(A) Have high glucose consumption
(B) Have high insulin production
(C) Have high mitotic rate
(D) Have short life span

214. Before FDG administration, the patient relaxes in a waiting room to minimize muscular activity, and in so doing minimizes any physiological uptake of FDG in the muscles. Hyperventilation may cause increased uptake in the:
    (A) The diaphragm
    (B) Leg muscles
    (C) Arm muscles
    (D) The peritoneum

215. Radioactive decay is the process by which an unstable atomic nucleus loses energy by emitting ionizing radiation. The emission is described as spontaneous meaning:
    (A) The nucleus decays without collision with another particle or atom
    (B) The nucleus decays after collision with another particle or atom
    (C) The nucleus decays without collision with shielding material
    (D) The nucleus decays after collision with shielding material

216. Brain natriuretic peptide (BNP) is 32 amino acid polypeptide secreted by the:
    (A) Brain
    (B) Heart
    (C) Kidney
    (D) Thyroid

217. A two-dimensional illustration of a three-dimensional allocation of the radiotracer in the myocardium which allows visualization of perfusion defects in a compressed format is known as:
    (A) Short axis display
    (B) Counts profile
    (C) Volume curve
    (D) Polar map

218. Side effects of the antithyroid medications include all of the following EXCEPT:
    (A) Agranulocytosis
    (B) Granulocytopenia
    (C) Aplastic anemia
    (D) Thrombocytosis

219. When tested Tc-99m sulfur colloid kit with TLC for free Tc-99m, the technologist noted: strip with free Tc-99m migrated to the solvent front reads 650 cpm, and strip containing Tc-99m sulfur colloid remaining at the point of origin reads 18350 cpm. What is the radiopharmaceutical impurity of this sulfur colloid kit?

    (A) 3%
    (B) 5%
    (C) 95%
    (D) 97%

220. The dose for cardiac first pass imaging studies must be contained in a volume not exceeding:

    (A) 0.5 ml
    (B) 1 ml
    (C) 2 ml
    (D) 3 ml

Answers

1. D – Right atrium (RA)

    Blood received by the right ventricle from the right atrium is propelled into the pulmonary artery and the pulmonary circulation. Oxygenated blood is returned by the pulmonary veins to the left atrium. The left ventricle ejects blood into systemic circulation.
    (Early and Sodee 1995)

2. C – Active transport

    Thyroid concentrates iodine from the blood stream in a gradient 20:1. The trapping mechanism operates through the Na^+/K^+ pump.
    (Early and Sodee 1995)

3. B – Ring artifacts

    If the counts in one pixel of the image are falsely decreased, then information at that location will be back-projected at the decreased level. The result in the reconstructed image will be a ring artifact, with the radius of the ring equal to the distance of that pixel from the COR.
    (O'Connor 2010)

4. D – Brain imaging

    Tc-99m sulfur colloid can also be used in esophageal transit time, gastroesophageal reflux, and gastric empty study.
    (Shackett 2008)

5. A – Hypokinetic left ventricle

    Hypokinesis – seen there on the anterior and apical surfaces – refers to decreased contractile function of the left ventricle, e.g., during a severe isch emia. The heart muscle in the distribution of the involved vessels is often hypokinetic due to the diminished blood supply.
    (Zaret and Beller 2005)

6. C – As Low as Reasonably Achievable

    It indicates making every reasonable attempt to maintain exposures to *ionizing radiation* as far below the dose limits as practical.
    (Saha 2004)

7. D – Provides good tissue penetration

    Tc-99m is a pure gamma emitter so no particle radiation is being produced; Tc-99m half-life is so long that body efficiently excretes it before it can have any real negative *health* effects.
    (Christian et al. 2004)

8. B –The hole at the top

   The dose calibrator is an ionization chamber used to determine the activity of radiopharmaceuticals. Once activity is detected (in a syringe or vial), the dose calibrator converts it – based on the radionuclide's gamma constant – to units of activity in curie or becquerel (Ci or Bq).
   (Early and Sodee 1995)

9. C – 1.7

   (Appendix A, Formula 10A)

10. A – The bone marrow

    Larger particles >100 nm accumulate in the liver and spleen.
    (Saha 2004)

11. C – Cardiac output

    The cardiac output (CO) is the stroke volume (SV) multiplied by the heart rate (HR) or $CO = SV \times HR$.
    (Early and Sodee 1995)

12. B – Lack of standardization

    Also, it is not an easy test, since the patient has to dry swallow for 10 min. The main indications for performing ES are to evaluate esophageal emptying and reflux in patients with esophageal dysmotility.
    (Odunsi and Camilleri 2009)

13. D – 662 keV gamma ray

    In larger amounts, Cs-137 is used in medical radiation therapy devices for treating cancer and in industrial gauges for detecting the flow of liquid through pipes.
    (Consultants in Nuclear Medicine)

14. D – Tachycardia

    Tachycardia is a rapid heart rate, usually defined as greater than 100 beats per minute.
    (Odunsi and Camilleri 2009)

15. C –The sinoatrial node

    Acting as the heart's natural pacemaker, the SA node (also commonly spelled sinuatrial node, abbreviated SA node or SAN, also called the sinus node) produces impulses at regular intervals to cause the heart to contract with a rhythm of about 60–70 beats per minute for a healthy, resting heart.
    (Podrid 2008)

16. C – Personnel monitoring

Misadministrations and sealed source inventory documentation should be kept for 5 years; 3 years of storage is required for patient dosage records.
(Early and Sodee 1995)

17. B – Bremsstrahlung radiation

Beta emitting substances should be shielded with low density materials, e.g., Plexiglas, plastic, wood because the rate of deceleration of the electron is slower and the radiation given off has a longer wavelength (less penetrating).
(Saha 2006)

18. A – Filtered backprojection

In the filtered backprojection (FBP) method – based on direct inversion of the Radon transform – the limited number of projections introduces streak artifacts in the image reconstructions.
(Christian 2004)

19. C – 0.00058 Ci

(Appendix A, Formula 9A)

20. A – Stress

Nonifectious inflammatory disease (NIID) e.g., vasculitis syndrome, granu-lomatous disorders, rheumatic fever can also induce fever.
(Bleeker-Rovers et al. 2009)

21. A – Give rescue breath

Occasional gasps, which can occur in the first minutes after sudden cardiac arrest (SCA), are not effective breaths.
(AHA Guidelines 2005)

22. D – Liver function

A Tc-99m methylene diphosphonate (Tc-99m MDP) is adsorbed onto the hydroxyapatite crystals on the mineralizing bone surfaces and kidney is the major route of radionuclide elimination.
(Gnanasegaran et al. 2009)

23. B – Detector and collimator

Extrinsic floods are performed with a collimator in place which allows evalu-ation of the particular collimator on the flood field.
(Early and Sodee 1995)

24. B – Body of scapulae

Tip of scapulae, acromioclavicular joint, and costochondral uptake are normal variants of the Tc-99m MDP bone scan of thoracic region.
(Gnanasegaran et al. 2009)

25. B – Static imaging

The specific imaging parameters, e.g., collimator type, time of acquisition, number of counts, matrix, etc. for a given exam will vary depending on the desired clinical information.
(Early and Sodee 1995)

26. C –Wearing film badge

Time, distance, and shielding are the three primary means of eliminating or reducing radiation exposures.
(Saha 2004)

27. C – Isobar

Isobars differ in *atomic number* (or number of *protons*) but not in *mass number*.
(Early and Sodee 1995)

28. D – The Constancy Test

The relative error test is used if only two observations are available; the chi-squared test is used with 10, 20, or more observations; the reliability factor is equal to the ratio of the sample standard deviation to the square root of the mean and is used with more than two observations.
(Lombardi 1999)

29. A – 4.8 mR/h

(Appendix A, Formula 16)

30. A – Thyroid and stomach

Other artifacts can be related to the patient, e.g., motion, prosthesis, radiotherapy, belt buckle, etc.
(Gnanasegaran et al. 2009)

31. C – Back pain

Some of the other symptoms of thyroid disease are: tachycardia, sensitivity to cold or heat, increased bowel movements or constipation, muscle weakness or spasms, moist or dry skin, irritability, sleep disturbances, fatigue, depression, and memory problems.
(Christian et al. 2004)

32. D – Lymph node(s)

It is important to document the site of injection in all patients to avoid confusion with bone abnormality.
(Gnanasegaran et al. 2009)

33. B – The byte

If the sequence contains eight bits, the word is referred to as a byte.
(Christian et al. 2004)

34. A – Active bleeding

Melena refers to the black, smelly, and tarry stool; hematemesis is the vomiting of blood and both conditions are signs of gastrointestinal bleeding.
(Howarth 2006)

35. A – Dynamic study

The time per frame should be decided on the temporal resolution needed for the study being performed. Quantitative studies require imaging time being sufficient enough with obtaining adequate statistics. For purposes of imaging only, longer times are generally preferred in order to provide sufficient image details.
(Early and Sodee 1995)

36. A – The critical organ

Target organ is the organ intended to receive the therapeutic dose of a radioactive substance.
(U.S. NRC Glossary 2010)

37. B – Radiotracer

One of the most important characteristics of a true radiotracer is the ability to study the components of a homeostatic system without disturbing their function.
(Vallabhajosula et al. 2010)

38. D – Linearity

The linearity test is performed at installation and quarterly. Actual measurements are matched up to expected measurements to determine if the instrument is linear throughout the activity range used in nuclear medicine department.
(Early and Sodee 1995)

39. B – 52%

(Appendix A, Formula 33)

40. D – Foreign body

Foreign body will be seen as a photopenic area and will not cause false-positive results.

(Howarth 2006)

41. D – Plain soaps cannot be contaminated

Nonantimicrobial soaps may be associated with substantial skin irritation and dryness. Trials have studied the effects of handwashing with plain soap and water vs., e.g., a chlorhexidine-containing detergent on healthcare-associated infection rates. Studies showed that healthcare-associated infection rates were lower when antiseptic handwashing was performed by personnel.

(CDC Guideline 2002)

42. A – Help to localize the site of bleeding

Static images may show blood in the gut that has already moved away from the actual site of bleeding.

(Howarth 2006)

43. D – Well counter and uptake probe

In the statistics of counting the chi-square test is used to find out whether there is a significant difference between the expected and the observed values in one or more categories.

(Early and Sodee 1995)

44. B – Small bowel

The small bowel is the longest portion of the gastrointestinal tract. It is much thinner when compared with the "large" bowel (colon), but it is much longer than the large bowel (14 ft on average).

(Howarth 2006)

45. B – (a) – anterior and (b) – posterior view

(Frohlich 2001)

46. D – Bioassay

Bioassays are also conducted to measure the effects of a given substance on a living *organism* and are crucial in the development of new *drugs* and in monitoring environmental *pollutants*.

(Saha 2004)

47. B – Radionuclide purity

The most common example radionuclide impurity is Mo-99 contaminant in Tc-99m radiopharmaceuticals.

(Saha 2006)

48. B – Photomultiplier tubes

    PMTs are light detectors: high internal gain makes the PMTs very sensitive devices.
    (Early and Sodee 1995)

49. C – 28 mR/h

    (Appendix A, Formula 17)

50. A – Block the capillaries in lungs

    Diameter of average capillary is 7 µm and the number of capillaries occluded compared to the total of 280 billion is almost negligible.
    (Saha 2004)

51. B – Chyme

    Chyle is a fluid consisting of a mixture of lymphatic fluid and chylomicrons that has a milky appearance.
    (Frohlich 1985)

52. C – Wall motion analysis

    Wall motion analysis is performed on processed single photon emission computed tomography (SPECT) myocardial perfusion images.
    (Zaret and Beller 2005)

53. D –Static, dynamic, and SPECT, images

    High count floods create uniformity correction matrix which is applied to all type of acquisitions performed on any given camera. Should be performed on monthly basis for at least 100 Mcts for each isotope used (vendor dependant).
    (Early and Sodee 1995)

54. D – Focal seizures

    Leukocytes are components of the blood. Changing patterns of bowel activity on delay images usually indicate distal passage of labeled granulocytes, or at times, bleeding within the bowel lumen.
    (Love and Palestro 2010)

55. D – 32

    A minimum of 16 frames per R–R interval are required for an accurate assessment of ventricular wall motion and assessment of ejection fraction. A higher framing rate (32–64 frames per R–R) allows for more precise end-systolic frame localization and is preferred for detailed measurement of diastolic filling parameters.
    (Zaret and Beller 2005)

56. C – Inverse square law

The inverse-square law applies not only to the physics of radiation – it is any *physical law* stating that some physical *quantity* or strength is *inversely proportional* to the *square* of the *distance* from the source of that physical quantity. (Early and Sodee 1995)

57. C – Potassium

Potassium is an essential dietary *mineral* and *electrolyte* and plays a key role in skeletal and smooth muscle contraction and is crucial to heart function. (Saha 2006)

58. C – The charcoal filter

Exhaled xenon is pulled through lead shielded traps filled with activated charcoal. Expended "U" shaped traps prolong the life of charcoal and provide a lengthy path for xenon runoff, allowing greater decay and absorption before exhaustion. Averaging 30–50 studies per month, the charcoal trap will last approximately 1 year. (Biodex 2010)

59. B – 6.4 h

(Appendix A, Formula 18)

60. C – Osteomyelitis

Osteomyelitis stimulates the uptake of leukocytes but suppresses the uptake of sulfur colloid. (Love and Palestro 2010)

61. A – Subcutaneous injection

Subcutaneous injections are given in small doses of 0.5–1 ml. Examples of subcutaneous administered medications include heparin, narcotics, allergy shots, etc. (Perry and Potter 2006)

62. C – Tc-99m SC is rapidly cleared from intravascular space

The Tc-99m tagged red blood cells (RBCs) have a stable presence within the blood pool, while the Tc-99m sulfur colloid (SC) as a blood pool agent is rapidly cleared-T1/2 of approximately 2–3 min – from intravascular space. As a result by 10–15 min after administration, SC has completely cleared from the blood pool into the liver, spleen, and, to a lesser degree, the bone marrow, while RBC activity is practically unchanged. (Howarth 2006)

63. A – Daily

The blank scan has been compared with the daily uniformity flood used for the gamma-camera.
(Saha 2005)

64. C – 2–3 min

As a result of rapid intravascular clearance 10–15 min after administration, SC has completely cleared from the blood pool into the liver, spleen, and, to a lesser extent, the bone marrow.
(Howarth 2006)

65. A – Normal scan

In normal circumstances, the regions of high stress, e.g., sacro-iliac joints or active growth appear as a "hot areas" when compared with the neighboring areas.
(Early and Sodee 1995)

66. D – Ventilation/perfusion scans

The advent of the new faster computed tomography (CT) scanners is responsible for shifting from nuclear medicine V/Q scans to the use of multidetector CT scans which are easier to read and are more specific.
(Mettler et al. 2008)

67. B – α, β, γ

The alpha particle consists of two protons and two neutrons, a beta particle is a high-velocity electron, and gamma rays are photons, not particles but the postemission products.
(Saha 2006)

68. D – Dose-calibrator linearity

In the decay method, 100–200 mCi of Technetium-99m in the glass vial is assayed. The time the measurement is taken and the activity are recorded. This same procedure is repeated at various time intervals for the next 36 h after the initial assay.

In the shield method, 100–200 mCi of Technetium-99m in the glass vial is assayed and the activity is recorded. In the next steps, the activity of the source vial is assayed in tube/tubes combinations and the measured activity is multiplied by the calibration factor for each of the tube/tubes combinations.
(Early and Sodee 1995)

69. A – 327,680 words

(Appendix A, Formula 24)

70. A – Lithogenic bile

Lithogenic bile favors gallstones production and may be associated with conditions like, e.g., increased secretion of *cholesterol* in the bile in obesity, high-caloric diets, etc.
(Wikipedia)

71. D – Height and weight

Many sources in the USA use blood glucose level and oxygen saturation as vital signs in addition to temperature, pulse, respiratory rate, and blood pressure. The other agencies include pupil size, equality, and reactivity to light or pain perceived by the patient to be vital sign as well.
(Kowalczyk and Donnett 1996)

72. D – Dose extravasation

The other mechanism other than cystic or common duct obstruction can be responsible for nonvisualization of gallbladder and resulting in false-positive studies, and include: parenteral nutrition (absence of oral intake), hepatocyte damage, decreased gallbladder contractility, etc.
(Ziessman 2009)

73. D – Allow greatly reduced injected radioactivity

The new imaging geometries using cadmium–zinc–telluride (CZT) detectors have higher sensitivity, higher energy, and higher spatial resolution which allow lowering the administered doses to the patient.
(ASNC Information Statement 2010)

74. B – Elevated alkaline phosphatase

The primary importance of measuring aspartate aminotransferase alkaline and alanine aminotransferase is to check the possibility of liver disease.
(Gnanasegaran et al. 2009)

75. C – Bone metastases

When cancer cells break away from a primary tumor, they can travel through the blood stream or lymph vessels to other parts of the body and lodge in an organ at a distant location (secondary tumor). Secondary tumors in the bone are called bone metastases.
(Christian et al. 2004)

76. D – Improving report turnaround time
(ASNC Information Statement 2010)

77. A – U.S. Pharmacopeia
(Saha 2006)

78. C – 6 months

The wipe sample must be taken from the nearest accessible point to the sealed source where contamination might accumulate.
(NRC 2000)

79. A – 126–154 keV

(Appendix A, Formula 22A)

80. B – Is determined by the method of sincalide infusion

Rapid sincalide infusions often cause nausea and cramps.
(Ziessman 2009)

81. D – The uterus

The uterus is a part of the genitourinary system or urogenital system which includes the *reproductive organs* and the *urinary system.*
(Frohlich 2001)

82. A – Reverse redistribution

(Zaret and Beller 2005)

83. C – Driver's name

A record of each shipment of licensed material should be kept for a period of 3 years after shipment.
(NRC 2004)

84. D – The right diaphragm

In patients diagnosed with Situs inversus totalis, the right diaphragm can cause the inferior wall defect.
(Zaret and Beller 2005)

85. B – Vertical long axis slices

In this view, the heart is in horizontal position and the apex of the heart is to the viewer's right. The tomogram is displayed with slices beginning at the septum and progressing to the lateral wall of the left ventricle.
(Zaret and Beller 2005)

86. D – Lung perfusion scan

Interventional fluoroscopically guided procedures may give fetal doses in the range of 10–100 mGy, X-ray of pelvis 1–4 mGy, CT of 8–49 mGy, and lung perfusion of 0.9 mGy.
(ICRP 2010)

87. B – Positron range

Greater path length results in a slight mispositioning of the annihilation event from the actual location of the positron-producing atom.

(Christian et al. 2004)

88. A – The light photons into an electrical signal

When a photon of sufficient energy hits the photocathode, it ejects a photoelectron which is accelerated toward dynodes. The amplification depends on the number of dynodes and the accelerating voltage; amplified electrical signal can be measured.

(Christian et al. 2004)

89. D – 8,500,000 rad

(Appendix A, Formula 9C)

90. B – Increase in false positive

Attenuation objects or structures can decreased counts density simulating presence of perfusion defect.

(Zaret and Beller 2005)

91. C – Phagocytosis

Phagocytosis is the process by which specialized macrophages, e.g., Kupffer cells, engulf and destroy microorganisms, and foreign bodies.

(Frohlich 2001)

92. C – Having a duration 500–1,500 ms

(Zaret and Beller 2005)

93. B – At low energy side of the energy window

Scattering of photons in matter results in a decrease in *energy* (increase in *wavelength*) of an *X-ray* or *gamma ray photon*.

(Early and Sodee 1995)

94. A – Reversible defect

(Zaret and Beller 2005)

95. C – Common bile duct

The common bile duct (CBD) is formed by the connection of the cystic duct that comes from the gallbladder and the common hepatic duct that comes from the liver. The CBD carries bile from the gallbladder and liver into the duodenum.

(Christian et al. 2004)

96. C – 50 rem/year
(Consultants in Nuclear Medicine 2010)

97. C – Decreased image resolution
(Christian et al. 2004)

98. B – Collimation
A collimator consists of a lead (Pb) plate containing a large number of small holes and is used to improve the spatial resolution of a gamma-camera.
(Early and Sodee 1999)

99. B – 18.7 mCi
(Appendix A, Formula 25)

100. B – Adenosine triphosphate
Adenosine triphosphate (ATP) is considered by biologists to be the energy currency of life. It is the high-energy molecule that stores the energy we need to do just about everything we do.
(Zaret and Beller 2005)

101. B – The lateral lobe
(Early and Sodee 1995)

102. B – False-negative studies
Methylxanthines is a common, naturally occurring group of stimulants. Caffeine, theophylline, and theobromine – the active ingredients of coffee, tea, cocoa, and cola beverages are in this group.
(Zaret and Beller 2005)

103. A – COR calibration
COR validation, not COR calibration, can be performed by the technologist.
(Halama 2010)

104. B – Be well hydrated
The patient should be well hydrated orally: 10 ml/kg of water or juice 30 min before imaging is recommended.
(Sfakianakis et al. 2009)

105. B – Grave's disease

Graves' disease – the most common cause of hyperthyroidism in the USA – is an autoimmune disorder in which the immune system makes thyroid-stimulating immunoglobulin that attaches to thyroid cells and mimics the action of thyroid-stimulating hormone (TSH).
(Early and Sodee 1995)

106. B – 0.002 rem in any 1 h

(Consultants in Nuclear Medicine 2010)

107. B – 0.693

$\lambda = 0.693/T_{1/2}$.
(Early and Sodee 1995)

108. B – Gas

A gas-filled tube usually with helium, neon, or argon briefly conducts an electrical current when a particle or photon of radiation temporarily ionizes the gas.
(Early and Sodee 1995)

109. C – 16.2 mCi

(Appendix A, Formula 25)

110. D – Meckel's diverticulum scan

A Tc-$99m$ pertechnetate scan is the procedure of choice to diagnose Meckel's diverticulum. Labeled white blood cells can be used in differential diagnosis of osteomyelitis.
(Early and Sodee 1995)

111. D – Dysphagia

Dyspepsia is defined as an uncomfortable feeling of epigastric discomfort, fullness, heartburn, bloating, etc. felt after eating.
(Mosby 1998)

112. C – Liver–spleen scan

No NPO required. A liver-spleen scintigraphy is useful in the diagnosis of hepatomegaly, splenomegaly, bone marrow shifting, tumors, lacerations, cysts, etc.
(Christian 2004)

113. A – Geiger-Mueller detector

The battery check and the sealed source check are performed daily by the nuclear medicine technologist to assess the sufficiency of the battery powering and the instrument sensitivity and consistency accordingly.
(Early and Sodee 1995)

114. A – Radioimmunotherapy

Radiotherapy and concurrent *chemotherapy* is called radiochemotherapy.
(Goldsmith 2010)

115. C – Obstructed pattern

Kidneys show gradually increasing activity with no response after Lasix administration.
(Christian 2004)

116. B – 18 or more years of age
(Nuclear Medicine Tutorials 2010)

117. B – Radionuclide

Radiopharmaceuticals have been defined as radioactive drugs that, when used for the purpose of diagnosis or therapy, typically elicit no physiological response from the patient.
(Early and Sodee 1995)

118. A – The physicist

Calibration is usually performed by the physicist who places the meter in front of a high-activity cesium sealed source producing exposure of at least 30 mR/h at 1 m. The exposure reading of the survey meter is calculated using the inverse square law and it should be adjusted to read the same (±10%) as the calculated value.
(Eradimaging 2010)

119. D – 62%
(Appendix A, Formula 34)

120. D – Performing pulmonary function tests

Medications interfering with MIBG uptake, e.g., reserpine, calcium channel blockers, or sympathomimetics have to be withdrawn in time.
(Grünwald and Ezziddin 2010)

121. C – The sinus node

Action potential from the sinus node spreads through the right and left atrium, reaches A–V node and after transmission through the bundle of His passes into the ventricular septum.

(Podrid 2008)

122. A – Mouse

"Ximabs" are the chimeric molecules and "zumabs" are the humanized molecules.

(Goldsmith 2010)

123. C – Battery check

Linearity, done quarterly, is also quality control procedure performed on the dose calibrator to assess the instrument's ability to measure accurately a range of low to high activities.

(Early and Sodee 1995)

124. B – A murine immunoglobulin is injected into a human

A mouse antibody injected to a human is recognized by the human *immune system* as a foreign protein (antigen). The human immune system then produces its own antibodies to fight the introduced mouse antibody (the HAMA response).

(Goldsmith 2010)

125. A – Growth plate

This uptake in epiphysis of the long bone is caused by hyperactive osteoblast due to child's growth. The quality of the bone scan can be judged by the sharpness of the appearance of the epiphyseal plates of the femora, tibiae, and fibulae.

(Christian et al. 2004)

126. D – Once a year

Although film badge readings are routinely posted on a monthly basis, every employer is responsible for informing each *employee* on an annual basis of his cumulative radiation dose.

(Nuclear Medicine Tutorials 2010)

127. A – Less mass than expected

(Early and Sodee 1995)

128. C – Geometry

Geometry warrants the ability of the instrument to accurately measure activities in different configured containers such as a syringes, vials, or pills.

(Early and Sodee 1995)

129. D – 46.6 mCi

(Appendix A, Formula 25)

130. D – Arrhythmias

Since a Y-90 Zevalin administration results in serious and prolonged cytopenias, the Zevalin therapeutic regimen should not be used to patients with significant marrow involvement and/or impaired bone marrow reserve.

(Goldsmith 2010)

131. D – Saliva

Most thromboemboli originate in the deep veins of the thigh. Stasis, hyperco-agulable state, and intimal injury are important factors in the development of thrombosis.

(Thompson and Hales 2010)

132. A – The reversibility of perfusion defects

(Zaret and Beller 2005)

133. B – Counter efficiency

Counter efficiency $= \text{cpm/dpm} \times 100$. The disintegrations per minute are cal-culated based on the activity of the source.

(Early and Sodee 1995)

134. B – The aggregation of the colloidal particles

A chelating agent (chelator) is a chemical that form complex molecules with certain metal ions so as to prevent ions from reacting with other ions or elements.

(Vallabhajosula et al. 2010)

135. B – Reversible defect

A defect that is present on the stress images and is not seen on the resting images is called reversible defect. Defect reversibility usually is a sign of myocardial ischemia. In our case, polar plot display indicates the presence of myocardial ischemia of the infero-basal wall.

(Christian et al. 2004)

136. C – Lukewarm area

The thyroid uptake room, the radioassay laboratory, and the computers room are examples of lukewarm areas. The cold areas are open to the public since no radioactivity is handled in these areas.

(Lombardi 1999)

137. B – Binding energy
(Early and Sodee 1995)

138. A – SPECT imaging
SPECT data can be acquired using step-and-shoot, continuous motion, or a hybrid technique, depending on the camera design and the type of study to be done and the COR is critical for this type of acquisition.
(Early and Sodee 1995)

139. D – 210 ml
(Appendix A, Formula 36A)

140. B – 0.08 mg/ml
A single-use vial or a single-use prefilled syringe injection solution containing regadenoson 0.4 mg/5 ml (0.08 mg/ml).
(Astellas 2010)

141. C – Ascending colon
The colon consists of four sections: the *ascending colon*, the *transverse colon*, the *descending colon*, and the *sigmoid colon*. The colon, the *cecum*, and the *rectum* make up the *large intestine*.
(Frohlich 1993)

142. D – Information whether the patient or a relative was notified
The licensee's name, the referring the brief description of the event, and the preventive action plan must be submitted. The patient's name must not be included in the report.
(Saha 2004)

143. D – Xenon leak test
The nebulizer does not necessitate any quality control procedure, but should be visually inspected for damage and cleaned when necessary.
(Early and Sodee 1995)

144. A – Oxidizes excess stannous ion
(Covidien 2010)

145. A – Repeat images after voiding
Having patient urinate reduces the bladder activity. If visualization of the pelvis is essential and patient is unable to void, bladder catheterization is indicated.
(Christian et al. 2004)

146. A – Warm area

The scanning room is an example of the warm area. The hot lab is an example of the hot area in the NM department where activities up to a few hundred millicuries may be stored and handled.
(Lombardi 1999)

147. C – Isomers

Isomer is any of two or more nuclides that consist of the same *number* of protons and the same number of neutrons but differ in energy.
(Saha 2004)

148. C – 25,000 cps

A point source centered over the detector guarantees a close to uniform photon flux striking on the detector.
(Zanzonico 2008)

149. A – 42 mCi

(Appendix A, Formula 25)

150. C – Package with expiration date August 1, 2011

(Early and Sodee 1995)

151. A – Atrioventricular septum

Atrioventricular septal defects are typically present in the fetal or neonatal period and are an important source of cardiac morbidity and mortality in this age group.
(Frohlich 1993)

152. D – Does not evaluate true thyroid function

Tc-99m although is being trapped by the thyroid cells is not being further organified as I-123.
(Christian et al. 2004)

153. B – Tc-99m, F-18, I-131

Energies of Co-57, Ba-133, and Ge-68 are 122 keV, 356 keV, and 511 keV, respectively. Compare their energies to that of Tc-99m (140 keV), 131I (364 keV), and 18F (511 keV).
(Zanzonico 2008)

154. B – Fine needle aspiration biopsy

A solitary "cold nodule" has a 5–10% probability of malignancy. Colloid cyst, abscess, nonfunctioning adenomas can also appear as a cold spots.
(Smith and Oates 2004)

155. A – Wrong labels

The first image on the left displays posterior view of pelvic, so it should be labeled " Lt Post Rt" not "Rt Post Lt." The second image from the left should be labeled "Lt Lat" and the third image should be labeled as "Rt Lat."
(Christian et al. 2004)

156. C – Promoting free radical production

Free radical damage may involve mitochondria, lysosomes, peroxisomes, nuclear endoplasmic reticulum, and plasma membranes. All of them are vital to the normal metabolic functions of the cell.
(Kassis 2008)

157. B – Lower energy, longer wavelength

Since the scattered X-ray photon has less energy, it has a longer wavelength and is less penetrating than the incident photon.
(Early and Sodee 1995)

158. B – Peaking linearity

The energy peak should be verified at least once a day to make sure that the photopeak is centered in the energy windows currently set.
(Early and Sodee 1995)

159. B – 2.64 ml

Answer of Formula 29 should be subtracted from the volume needed (3 ml) to get desired volume.
(Appendix A, Formulas 28A, 29)

160. B – Repeat images after water ingestion
(Smith and Oates 2004)

161. A – Thyroid

The heart, thymus, large vessels, lymph nodes, and connective tissue are also part of the mediastinum.
(Frohlich 1993)

162. D – Patient should use antiperspirant medications

A patient must also be instructed on how to reduce radiation exposure to the family and public members.
(SNM Guideline 2002)

163. B – 2, 2.5, 3, and 4 mm in width

The minimum perceptible bar spacing in a transmission image is used as an index of camera spatial resolution. All bars should appear straight (spatial linearity).
(Zanzonico 2008)

164. A – HIDA scan allows assessment of gallbladder function

A HIDA scan can be used to measure the rate at which bile is released from the gallbladder (gallbladder ejection fraction). Cholecystokinin (CCK) administration or standardized fatty meal consumption are the most commonly used interventions.
(Early and Sodee 1995)

165. B – Tc-99m sulfur colloid

Cerebral shunts are commonly used to treat *hydrocephalus*, due to excess buildup of *cerebrospinal fluid*. Shunt patency studies are performed to determine whether shunt revision surgery is needed in malfunctioned ventriculoperitoneal shunt.
(Christian et al. 2004)

166. B – Hypothyroidism

The only definite complication of RAI is a 1% incidence of radiation thyroiditis.
(Ross 2008)

167. B – Beta-particle emitters
(Kassis 2008)

168. B – Filtered backprojection and iterative techniques
(Christian et al. 2004)

169. D – 162 μCi
(Appendix A, Formula 31C)

170. B – Half-life

The biological half-life or elimination half-life of a substance is the time it takes for a *metabolite, drug*, radionuclide or other substance to lose half of its pharmacologic, physiologic, or radiologic activity.
(Mycek and Harvey 2008)

171. A – Infiltration
(Kozier and Erb 1993)

172. C – Continuous

The smaller the arc used for each projection, the less blurring from the camera motion.
(Christian et al. 2004)

173. C – Filtering
(Christian et al. 2004)

174. B – Atropine
Administration of atropine at the end of dobutamine infusion helps in achieving of 85% of aged predicted target heart rate (THR).
(Zaret and Beller 2005)

175. D – There is nothing wrong with these images
Liver–spleen images in Fig. 2.18 show normal homogeneous uptake of radiotracer in liver and spleen. Minor uptake of Tc-99m sulfur colloid is commonly seen in vertebrae and ribs during liver–spleen scan.
(Christian et al. 2004)

176. C – Wide
A specific license is given to the named persons for specific use of radioactive materials. General and broad licenses applied to, e.g., some laboratories and large medical centers accordingly.
(Halama 2010)

177. C – Neutrons and protons
A nucleon is a collective name for two particles: the *neutron* and the *proton* and they are components of the *atomic nucleus*. The nucleons are made of three *quarks*.
(Christian et al. 2004)

178. A – Material Safety Data Sheet (MSDS)
In the *USA*, the *Occupational Safety and Health Administration* (OSHA) requires that MSDS be available to employees for potentially harmful substances handled in the workplace.
(OSHA 1994)

179. C – 0.37 min
When there is huge difference between the biological half-life and the physical half-life, shorter of both becomes the effective half-life.
(Appendix A, Formula 18)

180. C – Radium 223
The alpha emitter radium-223 is a bone-seeking radionuclide studied as a novel treatment for patients with bone metastases. Ra-223 showed minimal toxicity in a phase 1 study.
(Saha 2004)

181. C – The medium lobe

The right lobe, the left lobe, the caudate lobe, and the quadrate lobe are the four lobes of the liver.
(Frohlich 1993)

182. B – Infection

An infection is defined as an invasion and multiplying of pathogens – certain bacteria, viruses, fungi, and parasites – in the body tissues in which they are not usually present.
(Bleeker-Rovers et al 2009)

183. B – Apex

The apical slices are displayed first with progression toward the cardiac base with the superior plane at the top and the inferior at the bottom.
(Zaret and Beller 2005)

184. B – Injected dose
(Lin and Alavi 2009)

185. B – Parathyroid

Note the uptake in salivary glands and the heart visualization – lower left corner – due to Tc-99m sestamibi uptake in the myocardium.
(Christian et al. 2004)

186. B – The Radiation Safety Officer (RSO)
(Radiologyinfo.org 2010)

187. D – Pain in bony metastases

Two radiopharmaceuticals: strontium-89 (Metastron) and samarium-153 (Quadramet) can be used for the treatment of painful skeletal metastases (e.g., bone metastases from prostate cancer, breast cancer, or any other cancer that metastasizes to the bone).
(Christian et al. 2004)

188. B – Increased sensitivity and decreased resolution

Increase the thickness of the scintillation detector will increase γ-ray absorption; however, increased thickness will result in more Compton scattering causing degradation of resolution.
(Saha 2006)

189. A – 95.3 μCi

(Appendix A, Formula 30A)

190. D – Delay imaging is performed
   (Lin and Alavi 2009)

191. D – Decreased appetite
   The blend of weight loss and increased appetite is a characteristic finding in patients with evident hyperthyroidism; however, some patients gain weight, especially younger ones due to the excessive appetite stimulation.
   (Andreoli et al. 2001)

192. A – Myelosuppression
   P-32 therapy has not been accepted commonly because of its known bone marrow toxicity.
   (Saha 2004)

193. C – Display monitor
   (Early and Sodee 1995)

194. A – Sinogram
   A sinogram has all the projection information necessary to reconstruct a single slice of the original activity allocation.
   (Christian et al. 2004)

195. B – Anterior
   Since the heart is located anterior to the lung, it projects greatest shadow in the anterior view.
   (Christian et al. 2004)

196. C – Rems
   The curie and becquerel measure the amount of radioactivity; the rad is the measure of absorbed dose.
   (Early and Sodee 1995)

197. C – Are used for radionuclide therapy
   (Kassis 2008)

198. A – Decrease
   An increased volume of the sample will result in more count "escaping" the detector through the well counter opening.
   (Saha 2006)

199. C – 32%
   (Appendix A, Formula 38A)

200. A – Transient Ischemic Dilation

TID is most likely caused by stress-induced ischemia to the innermost layer of the ventricle.
(Zaret and Beller 2005)

201. A – Millimeters of mercury
(Kowalczyk and Donnett 1996)

202. A – Free of superimposition
(Ziessman 2009)

203. C – Accuracy
(Early and Sodee 1995)

204. B – The same number of beats
(Zaret and Beller 2005)

205. B – Right nephrectomy

Unusual findings might be nonsignificant or incidental, such as dextrocardia, liver cysts, postmastectomy changes but occasionally these findings may require further evaluation as they may indicate an unexpected malignancy, e.g., breast or lung carcinoma. The raw projection images should always be reviewed for any unusual findings, as well as for potential causes of image artifacts.
(Zaret and Beller 2005)

206. C – Patient undergoing NM study with radiopharmaceutical administration
(Early and Sodee 1995)

207. C – Gamma photons
(Early and Sodee 1995)

208. C – Contact
(Early and Sodee 1995)

209. B – 1.5 mm

Simple way to solve this type of problem is by dividing the given exposure rate by 2 until desired exposure rate is achieved. Each division by 2 represents one HVL, since exposure is reduced to half. If you divide initial exposure rate by two 7 times, then you have gone through 7 HVLs to achieve desired exposure rate. To obtain answer just multiply the amount of HVLs by the HVL of a given isotope (7×0.21).
(Appendix A, Formula 17)

210. B – Hepatobiliary tract

Thirty-three percentage of the injected dose is excreted through the hepatobiliary tract and 25% through the kidneys.
(Christian 2004)

211. B – Free fatty acids

The myocardium can use different substrates according to their availability, hormonal status, and other factors. In a typical fasting state, the myocardium primarily utilizes free fatty acids, but after a meal or a glucose load, it prefers glucose.
(Christian 2004)

212. C – Tc-99m MIBI washes out more rapidly from the thyroid than from abnormal parathyroid

The retention of tracer in abnormal parathyroid is related to the presence of rich in mitochondria oxyphil cells.
(Palestro et al. 2005)

213. A – Have high glucose consumption

High spatial resolution and rapid accumulation into inflammation foci are major benefits of PET FDG over conventional imaging.
(Lin and Alavi 2009)

214. A – The diaphragm
(Lin and Alavi 2009)

215. A – The nucleus decays without collision with another particle or atom
(Wikipedia 2010)

216. B – *Heart*

BNP belongs to a family of protein hormones called natriuretic peptides. BNP acts on blood vessels, causing them to widen and on the kidneys promoting salt and water excretion.
(Family Health Guide 2010)

217. D – Polar map

Circumferential profiles generated from the short axis slices are normalized to the reference area in the rest or stress study. The rest or stress is subtracted from the normalized data, and then displayed as a polar bull's-eye plot so that positive values show areas that have "reverse" or "improved." Patient profiles are compared with means and standard deviations of reversibility for all pixels determined from the database of normal files.
(Zaret and Beller 2005)

218. D – Thrombocytosis

Thrombocytosis is the presence of high *platelet* counts in the *blood* – often symptomless but it can predispose to *thrombosis* in some patients. (Andreoli et al. 2001)

219. A – 3%

(Appendix A, Formula 32B)

220. B – 1 ml

(Zaret and Beller 2005)

References and Suggested Readings

American Heart Association Guidelines for Cardiopulmonary Resuscitation and Emergency Cardiovascular Care. Circulation. http://circ.ahajournals.org/cgi/content/full/112/24_suppl/IV-47. Accessed 11 Apr 2007.

Andreoli TE, Bennett JC, et al. Cecil essentials of medicine. 5th ed. Philadelphia, PA: WB Saunders Company; 2001.

ASNC Information Statement. Recommendations for reducing radiation exposure in myocardial perfusion imaging. http://www.asnc.org/imageuploads/RadiationReduction060110.pdf. Accessed 23 Aug 2010.

Astellas. http://www.lexiscan.com/about/about.php. Accessed 5 Sept 2010.

Biodex. Pulmonex II® Xenon System. http://www.biodex.com/radio/lungvent/lung_502feat.htm. Accessed 17 Nov 2010.

Bleeker-Rovers CP, Van der Meer JW, Oyen WJ. Fever of unknown origin. Semin Nucl Med. 2009;39:81–7.

Braunwald L et al. Harrison's principles of internal medicine. 15th ed. New York, NY: McGraw-Hill; 2001.

CDC. Guideline for hand hygiene in health-care settings. http://www.cdc.gov/mmwr/PDF/rr/rr5116.pdf. Accessed 21 June 2010.

Christian PE, Bernier DR, Langan JK. Nuclear medicine and PET. Technology and techniques. 5th ed. St. Louis, MO: Mosby; 2004.

Covidien. Technescan. MAG3 Kit for the preparation of Technetium Tc-99m mertiatide. Package insert. 2010.

Early PJ, Sodee BD. Principles and practice of nuclear medicine. 2nd ed. St. Louis, MO: Mosby; 1995.

Eradimaging. Nuclear Medicine Instrumentation and quality control: a review. http://eradimaging.com/site/article.cfm?ID=88&mode=ce. Accessed 28 Oct 2010.

Family Health Guide. Harvard Medical School. http://www.health.harvard.edu/fhg/updates/BNP-An-important-new-cardiac-test.shtml. Accessed 22 Sept 2010.

Frohlich ED. Rypin's basic sciences review. 18th ed. Philadelphia, PA: J.B. Lippincott Company; 2001.

Gnanasegaran G, Gary CG, Adamson K, Fogelman I. Patterns, variants, artifacts, and pitfalls in conventional radionuclide bone imaging and SPECT/CT. Semin Nucl Med. 2009;39:380–95.

Goldsmith SJ. Radioimmunotherapy of lymphoma: Bexxar and Zevalin. Semin Nucl Med. 2010;40:122–35.

Grünwald F, Ezziddin S. 131I-Metaiodobenzylguanidine therapy of neuroblastoma and other neuroendocrine tumors. Semin Nucl Med. 2010;40:153–63.

Halama RJ. Radiation safety, radiopharmacy, instrumentation and physics. 13th Annual nuclear medicine review course. Consultants in nuclear Medicine. 2010;08/30 Sept 2001.

Howarth DM. The role of nuclear medicine in the detection of acute gastrointestinal bleeding. Semin Nucl Med. 2006;36:133–46.

ICRP. Pregnancy and medical radiation. http://www.icrp.org/downloadDoc.asp?document=docs/ICRP_84. Accessed 14 Aug 2010.

Karesh P. Consultants in nuclear medicine. http://www.nucmedconsultants.com. Accessed 7 June 2010.

Kassis AI. Therapeutic radionuclides. Biophysical and radiobiologic principles. Semin Nucl Med. 2008;38:358–66.

Kowalczyk N, Donnett K. Integrated patient care for the imaging professionals. St. Louis, MO: Mosby; 1996.

Kozier B, Erb G. Techniques in clinical nursing. 4th ed. Redwood City, CA: Addison-Wesley; 1993.

Lin CE, Alavi A. PET and PET/CT. A clinical guide. 2nd ed. New York, NY: Thieme; 2009.

Lombardi MH. Radiation safety in nuclear medicine. Boca Raton, FL: CRC Press LLC; 1999.

Love C, Palestro CJ. Altered biodistribution and incidental findings on gallium and labeled leukocyte/bone marrow scans. Semin Nucl Med. 2010;40(4):271–82.

Mettler FA, Bhargavan M, et al. Nuclear medicine exposure in the United States, 2005–2007: preliminary results. Semin Nucl Med. 2008;38(5):384–91.

Mettler FA, Guiberteau MJ. Essentials of nuclear medicine imaging. 5th ed. Philadelphia, PA: Saunders Elsevier; 2006.

Mosby's Medical, Nursing & Allied Health Dictionary. 5th ed. St. Louis, MO: Mosby; 1998.

Mycek MJ, Harvey RA. Lippincott's illustrated reviews: pharmacology. 3rd ed. Philadelphia, PA: Lippincott; 2008.

Nuclear Medicine Tutorials. http://www.nucmedtutorials.com/index.html. Accessed 7 June 2010.

O'Connor MK. Quality control of scintillation cameras (Planar and SPECT). http://www.aapm.org/meetings/99AM/pdf/2741-51264.pdf. Accessed 25 Sept 2010.

Odunsi ST, Camilleri M. Selected interventions in nuclear medicine: gastrointestinal motor functions. Semin Nucl Med. 2009;39:186–94.

OSHA. United States Department of Labor. http://www.osha.gov/. Accessed 10 Sept 2009.

Palestro JC, Tomas BM, Tronco GG. Radionuclide imaging of the parathyroid glands. Semin Nucl Med. 2005;35:266–76.

Perry AG, Potter PA. Clinical nursing skills and techniques. 7th ed. St. Louis, MO: Mosby Elsevier; 2006.

Pitman KT. Sentinel node localization in head and neck tumors. Semin Nucl Med. 2005;35:253–6.

Podrid PJ. ECG tutorial. Official reprint from UpToDate. http://www.uptodate.com. Accessed 5 May 2008.

Radiologyinfo. http://www.radiologyinfo.org/. Accessed 10 Sept 2010.

Ross SD. Radioiodine in the treatment of hyperthyroidism. Official reprint from UpToDate. http://www.uptodate.com. Accessed 2 Oct 2008.

Saha GB. Basics of PET imaging. New York, NY: Springer; 2005.

Saha GB. Fundamentals of nuclear pharmacy. 5th ed. New York, NY: Springer; 2004.

Saha GB. Physics and radiobiology of nuclear medicine. 3rd ed. New York, NY: Springer; 2006.

Sfakianakis G, Sfakianaki E, Georgiu M, et al. A renal protocol for all ages and all indications: mercapto-acetyl-triglycine (MAG3) with simultaneous injection of Furosemide (MAG3-F0): a 17-year experience. Semin Nucl Med. 2009;39(3):156–73.

Shackett P. Nuclear medicine technology: procedure and quick reference. 2nd ed. Philadelphia, PA: Lippincott Williams & Wilkins; 2008.

Smith J, Oates E. Radionuclide imaging of the thyroid gland: patterns, pearls, and pitfalls. Clin Nucl Med. 2004;29:181–93.

SNM. Procedure guideline for therapy of thyroid disease with iodine-131. J Nucl Med. 2002;43(6):856–61.

Stein PD, Woodard PK, Weg JG, et al. Diagnostic pathways in acute pulmonary embolism: recommendations of the PIOPED II investigators. Radiology. 2007;242:15–21.

Thompson BT, Hales CA. Overview of acute pulmonary embolism. Official reprint from UpToDate. http://www.uptodate.com. Accessed 15 July 2010.

U.S. NRC. Glossary. http://www.nrc.gov/reading-rm/basic-ref/glossary/critical-organ.html. Accessed 26 Sept 2010.

U.S. NRC. Leak testing of sealed sources. http://www.nrc.gov/reading-rm/doc-collections/cfr/part039/part039-0035.html. Accessed 15 Sept 2010.

U.S. NRC. Procedures for receiving and opening packages. http://www.nrc.gov/reading-rm/doc-collections/cfr/part020/part020-1906.html. Accessed 3 Sept 2010.

Vallabhajosula S, Killeen R, Osborne J. Altered biodistribution of radiopharmaceuticals: role of radiochemical/pharmaceutical purity, physiological, and pharmacologic factors. Semin Nucl Med. 2010:40:220–41.

Wikipedia. Basic physics of nuclear medicine/computers in nuclear medicine. http://en.wikipedia.org/wiki. Accessed 19 June 2010.

Zanzonico P. Routine quality control of clinical nuclear medicine instrumentation: a brief review. J Nucl Med. 2008;49:1114–31.

Zaret BL, Beller GA. Clinical nuclear cardiology: state of the art and future directions. 3rd ed. Philadelphia, PA: Mosby; 2005.

Ziessman H. Interventions used with cholescintigraphy for the diagnosis of hepatobiliary disease. Semin Nucl Med. 2009;39:174–85.

Chapter 3
Practice Test #2: Difficulty Level – Moderate*

Questions

1. Which of the following statements regarding the use of "cough cardiopulmo-nary resuscitation (CPR)" is TRUE?
   (A) Cough CPR is useful for the treatment of unresponsive victim
   (B) Coughing does not generates blood flow to the brain
   (C) Coughing helps maintain consciousness
   (D) Cough CPR should be taught to lay rescuers

2. Atropine is an anticholinergic agent frequently used with dobutamine stress testing to increase:
   (A) Blood pressure
   (B) Heart rate
   (C) Oxygen supply
   (D) Vasospasm

3. The ratio of net counts in the photopeak to net counts in the entire spectrum is called:
   (A) Photopeak efficiency
   (B) Photopeak window
   (C) Energy resolution
   (D) Energy constant

*Answers to Test #2 begin on page 131.

A. Moniuszko and D. Patel, *Nuclear Medicine Technology Study Guide: A Technologist's*   83
Review for Passing Board Exams, DOI 10.1007/978-1-4419-9362-5_3,
© Springer Science+Business Media, LLC 2011

4. Patients with compromised renal function and referred for renal scintigraphy with Lasix will receive the dose of diuretic that:
   (A) Should be decreased
   (B) Should be increased
   (C) Should not be changed
   (D) Should be doubled

5. Figure 3.1 presents the schematic drawing of normal heart conduction system. The label "b" represents:
   (A) The left bundle branch
   (B) The right bundle branch
   (C) The sinoatrial node
   (D) The atrioventricular node

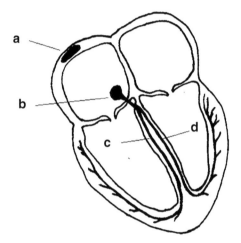

Fig. 3.1 Schematic drawing of normal heart conduction system (*Illustration by Sabina Moniuszko*)

6. The majority of radiation exposure to personnel performing PET/CT procedures comes from the:
   (A) PET scanner
   (B) CT scanner
   (C) Injected patient
   (D) Unopened dose pig

7. The system of units that officially came into being in October 1960 and has been adopted by nearly all countries is known by all of the following names EXCEPT:
   (A) Universal System
   (B) Systeme Internationale (S.I.)
   (C) Metric System
   (D) International System

8. The process that resets a Geiger–Müller survey meter to its normal, ready to detect another particle state, is known as:
   (A) Quenching
   (B) Depolarization
   (C) Pitching
   (D) Calibration

9. 3.4 curies (Ci) is equal to:
   (A) 0.0000034 microcurie (μCi)
   (B) 0.0034 microcurie (μCi)
   (C) 3,400 microcuries (μCi)
   (D) 3,400,000 microcuries (μCi)

10. Obstruction in the airways should be seen as a hot spot on the ventilation Xe-133 scan:
   (A) In washout phase
   (B) In equilibrium phase
   (C) In single breath phase
   (D) In all phases

11. The majority of antiseptics used in hand-washing are alcohol-based antiseptics. Which of the following statements describes correctly theirs properties?
   (A) The antimicrobial activity of alcohols can be attributed to their ability to inhibit protein synthesis
   (B) Alcohol solutions containing 100% alcohol are most effective
   (C) Alcohols have poor in vitro germicidal activity against gram-positive and gram-negative vegetative bacteria
   (D) Alcohols are rapidly germicidal when applied to the skin, but they have no appreciable persistent activity

12. The sympathetic nervous system has great influence on cardiovascular physiology and is responsible for regulating myocardial blood flow, heart rate, and the contractile performance of the heart. Which of the following radiotracers can be used for imaging the sympathetic nervous system of the heart?
    (A) I-123 metaiodobenzylguanidine (MIBG)
    (B) I-131 iodoamphetamine (IMP)
    (C) I-125 human serum albumin (RISA)
    (D) Tc-99m hexamethylpropyleneamine oxime (HMPAO)

13. The ratio of radiations striking the detector divided by the total number of radiations produced by the source is called:
    (A) Photopeak efficiency
    (B) Geometric efficiency
    (C) Energy resolution
    (D) Energy window

14. Recent consensus guidelines for Scintigraphic Gastric Emptying known as A Joint Report of The Society of Nuclear Medicine (SNM) and The American Neurogastroenterology and Motility Society (ANMS), recommends a standardized low-fat egg-white meal and images taken at:
    (A) 0, 1, 2, and 4 h
    (B) 0, 1, 3, and 4 h
    (C) 0, 1, 2, 3, and 4 h
    (D) 0, 2, 3, and 4 h

15. Figure 3.2 presents the diagrams of end-systolic (dashed line) and end-diastolic (solid line) shape of left ventricle cineangiogram. The drawing "a" represents normal left ventricle wall motion. What left ventricle abnormality corresponds to the drawing "b"?
    (A) Hypokinetic left ventricle
    (B) Hyperkinetic left ventricle
    (C) Akinetic left ventricle
    (D) Dyskinetic left ventricle

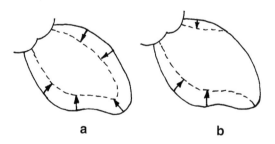

a   b

Fig. 3.2 End-systolic (dashed line) and end-diastolic (solid line) shape of left ventricle cineangiogram (*Illustration by Sabina Moniuszko*)

16. US population total exposure to ionizing radiation has nearly doubled over the past two decades, a rise largely attributed to increase exposure from:
    (A) Frequent flying
    (B) Diagnostic imaging
    (C) Natural background radiation
    (D) Nuclear reactors

17. Which of the following sentences correctly describes a positron?
    (A) A particle having a mass equal to the proton and no charge
    (B) A particle having a mass equal to the proton but opposite charge
    (C) A particle having a mass equal to the electron but opposite charge
    (D) A particle having a mass equal to the electron and no charge

18. Statistics of counting errors due to carelessness and/or lack of knowledge, or negligence are called:
    (A) Random errors
    (B) Blunders
    (C) Systematic errors
    (D) Deviation errors

19. 24 h post oral radioiodine administrations following counts were obtained from the thyroid gland: 32,829, 33,103, and 32,940. What is the standard deviation of the obtained counts?
    (A) 108
    (B) 114
    (C) 124
    (D) 138

20. All of the following scintigraphic methods are often used in the diagnosis of fever of unknown origin (FUO) EXCEPT:
    (A) Fluorodeoxyglucose-positron emission tomography (FDG-PET)
    (B) Ga-67 citrate scintigraphy
    (C) Labeled leukocytes scintigraphy
    (D) Labeled erythrocytes scintigraphy

21. The rate of gastric emptying is controlled primarily by reflexes that occur:
    (A) During swallowing
    (B) During chewing
    (C) When chyme enters the stomach
    (D) When chyme enters the intestine

22. The bone scan is one of the most common diagnostic procedures performed in nuclear medicine. Radionuclide bone scintigraphy is characterized by:
    (A) High sensitivity and low specificity
    (B) High sensitivity and high specificity
    (C) Low sensitivity and low specificity
    (D) Low sensitivity and high specificity

23. A QC test performed in nuclear medicine department to assess the reproducibility of radiation counter if only two observations are available is called:
    (A) The relative error
    (B) The chi-squared test
    (C) The reliability factor
    (D) The constancy test

24. A linear display of rib lesions in adjacent ribs seen on the bone scintigraphy is typical for:
    (A) Metastatic lesions
    (B) Fracture with history of trauma
    (C) Paget's disease
    (D) Osteomyelitis

25. Figure 3.3 presents the schematic coronary tree diagram. Right coronary artery supplies:
    (A) Septal portion of the heart
    (B) Inferior portion of the heart
    (C) Anterior portion of the heart
    (D) Posterior portion of the heart

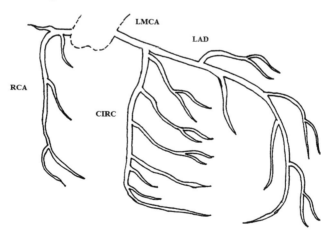

Fig. 3.3 Schematic coronary tree diagram (*Illustration by Sabina Moniuszko*)

26. The radiation dose for the patient referred for the bone scan imaging and receiving 10 mCi of F-18 fluoride is higher than radiation dose for the patient receiving 25 mCi of Tc-99m methylene diphosphonate (MDP). Which of the following statements adequately compares those two exposures?
    (A) Tc-99m MDP exposure is half of F-18 fluoride
    (B) Radiation exposures are almost equal
    (C) F-18 fluoride exposure is 70% higher than Tc-99m
    (D) Tc-99m MDP exposure is ten times smaller than F-18

27. The mass of a beta particle is essentially the same as the mass of:
    (A) An electron
    (B) An alpha particle
    (C) A proton
    (D) A neutrino

28. A volatile form of memory used for the short-term storage of information is called:
    (A) Random Access Memory (RAM)
    (B) Read Only Memory (ROM)
    (C) Central Processing Unit (CPU)
    (D) Digital-to-Analog Converter (DAC)

29. The following results were obtained from 5-year-old child's voiding cystogram study:
    – Voided urine volume – 103 ml
    – Pre-void counts – 135,324
    – Post-void counts – 35,523

    What is the child's bladder residual volume?
    (A) 36.7 ml
    (B) 42.2 ml
    (C) 46.3 ml
    (D) 53.7 ml

30. Transient increase in tracer uptake in responding metastases in the early months after chemotherapy/hormone therapy for breast and prostate cancer is called:
    (A) Super scan
    (B) Flare phenomenon
    (C) Super phenomenon
    (D) Flare scan

31. Oxygenated blood from the lungs enters the right atrium via:
    (A) Pulmonary artery
    (B) Pulmonary veins
    (C) Aorta
    (D) Superior vena cava

32. A bone scan is used for evaluating the skeletal system. Extraosseus, pulmonary uptake on bone scintigraphy can be seen in patients with:
    (A) Radiation pneumonitis
    (B) Emphysema
    (C) Pneumothorax
    (D) Viral pneumonia

33. The correlation between the number of counts and display intensity is commonly linear which provides uniform shading between all counts intensities. A logarithmic relationship between the number of counts and display intensity:
    (A) Suppresses low counts
    (B) Reduces the low count pixels
    (C) Enhances low counts
    (D) Expends the number of shades in the high pixel values

34. Confirmatory tests for the adult brain death may include all of the following EXCEPT:
    (A) Electroencephalography-electrical activity
    (B) Contrast angiography-blood flow
    (C) Transcranial Doppler ultrasound-blood flow
    (D) Magnetic resonance imaging-magnetic activity

35. Static images presented in Fig. 3.4 are frequently obtained to evaluate the hepatobiliary tract. What was the dose and what radiopharmaceutical was used in this procedure?
    (A) 25.4 mCi of Tc-99m Methylene diphosphonate
    (B) 10.4 mCi of Tc-99m Tagged RBCs
    (C) 6.2 mCi of Tc-99m Sulfur colloid
    (D) 5.9 mCi of Tc-99m Mebrofenin

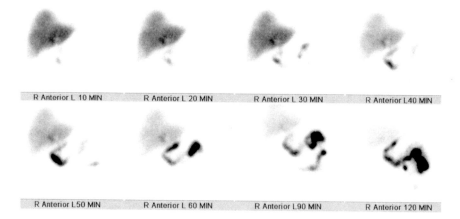

Fig. 3.4 Static images of the hepatobiliary tract

36. Available data on the number of nuclear medicine examinations performed between 1972 through 2005 shows a marked shift in the type of procedures performed. During this period:
    (A) The number of performed brain and thyroid studies increased
    (B) The number performed of cardiac imaging procedures increased
    (C) The number of performed bone scans increased
    (D) The number of performed V/Q scans increased

37. Nuclides with the same mass and atomic number, but with different energy levels are known as:
    (A) Isomers
    (B) Isotopes
    (C) Isobars
    (D) Isotones

38. The system that can control the memory system for reading and/or writing independently of the Central Processing Unit (CPU) is called:
    (A) Digital-to-Analog Converter (DAC)
    (B) Lookup Table (LUT)
    (C) Analog-to-Digital Converter (ADC)
    (D) Direct memory access (DMA)

39. 780 Sv (sieverts) is equal to how many rem/s (roentgen equivalent man)?
    (A) 78,000 rems
    (B) 780 rems
    (C) 0.078 rem
    (D) 0.00078 rem

40. Tc-99m-labeled sulfur colloid gastrointestinal bleeding scintigraphy:
    (A) Allows delayed 24 h imaging
    (B) Is characterized by rapid blood clearance
    (C) Is time consuming due to the dose preparation procedure
    (D) Allows rapid identification of bleeding site from stomach

41. Control of synthesis and secretion of thyroid hormones by thyroid-stimulating hormone (TSH) secreted by pituitary gland is maintained by mechanism called:
    (A) Supervision
    (B) Negative Feedback
    (C) Ruling
    (D) Positive Response

42. The number of positive gastrointestinal bleeding scans in published series range from 26 to 82%. This wide variation of results largely reflects:
    (A) Interpretative skills
    (B) Patients gender
    (C) Patients selection
    (D) Imaging protocols

43. Well Counter (WC) and Uptake Probe (UP) are two detectors commonly configured to a single computer. Which of the following statements describing their properties is INCORRECT?
    (A) WC counts patient samples, UP counts activity within the patient
    (B) They are solid sodium iodide crystal detectors
    (C) WC counts activity within the patient, UP counts patient samples
    (D) They measure activity in units of counts or counts per minute

44. Pathologic Tc-99m methylene diphosphonate (MDP) breast uptake should be differentiated from normal physiological uptake. The physiological Tc-99m uptake can be described by all of the following EXCEPT:
    (A) Is generally symmetric
    (B) Is mild
    (C) Is often seen in the young postpubescent population
    (D) Is misinterpreted as breast attenuation artifact

45. Images Fig. 3.5 were acquired during routine lung perfusion scintigraphy and they should be labeled:
    (A) a- and b-posterior views
    (B) a-posterior and b-anterior view
    (C) a-anterior and b-posterior view
    (D) a- and b-anterior views

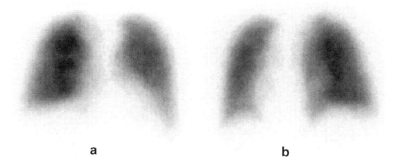

a   b

Fig. 3.5 Lung perfusion scintigraphy

46. The dosimetric quantity useful for comparing the overall health effects of irradiation of the whole body, which takes into account the absorbed doses received by various organs and tissues, is called:
    (A) Effective dose
    (B) Whole body dose
    (C) Dose coefficient
    (D) Dose equivalent

47. One of the most common problems associated with radiopharmaceuticals is an altered biodistribution. All of the following can affect the normal radiopharmaceutical biodistribution EXCEPT:
    (A) Drug interactions
    (B) Previous medical procedures
    (C) Route of radiopharmaceutical administration
    (D) Procedure type

48. Linearity of the scintillation gamma camera is performed to assess the acquired images for:
    (A) Horizontal and vertical line straightness
    (B) Reproducibility with different isotopes used
    (C) Resolution
    (D) Contrast

49. Tl-201 has physical half-life of 73 h and biological half-life of 10 days. What is the effective half-life of Tl-201?
    (A) 55 h
    (B) 48 h
    (C) 40 h
    (D) 35 h

50. Radiolabeled urine may enter the bowel and lead to intense visualization of affected bowel segments when:
    (A) Fistulous connection is present
    (B) Dose was extravasated
    (C) Contamination was present
    (D) Patient moved during the scan

51. The adrenal medulla is typically located within the adrenal gland surrounded by the adrenal cortex. The adrenal medulla synthesizes and secretes:
    (A) Catecholamines
    (B) Androgens
    (C) Estrogens
    (D) Mineralocorticoids

52. Routine display of the raw projection myocardial perfusion images allows discovery of incidental findings. Hepatic cyst will present as:
    (A) Hot area
    (B) Photopenic area
    (C) Attenuation artifact
    (D) Motion artifact

53. All of the following quality control procedures are necessary for a general nuclear medicine cameras proper functioning EXCEPT:
    (A) Energy peaking, collimator integrity, and uniformity
    (B) Efficiency, resolution, and linearity
    (C) High calibration flood, collimator integrity, and efficiency
    (D) Reproducibility, uniformity, and blank scan

54. Tc-99m- and In-111-labeled leukocyte imaging (WBC) are established procedures for diagnosing inflammation and infection. All of the following wounds appear as areas of intense activity on WBC images EXCEPT:
    (A) Skin grafts wounds
    (B) Surgical incision wounds
    (C) Ileostomies wounds
    (D) Tracheostomies wounds

55. Presented images, Fig. 3.6 were acquired during the procedure frequently use to evaluate hepatosplenomegaly. What were the dose and radiopharmaceutical used in this of procedure?
    (A) 25.1 mCi of Tc-99m Sulfur colloid
    (B) 12.1 mCi of Tc99m Mebrofenin
    (C) 6.1 mCi of Tc-99m Sulfur colloid
    (D) 1.1 mCi of Tc-99m Mebrofenin

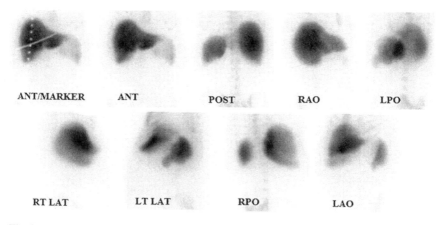

ANT/MARKER   ANT   POST   RAO   LPO

RT LAT   LT LAT   RPO   LAO

Fig. 3.6 Liver-spleen scintigraphy

56. Absorbed and effective dose to a patient will increase if patient is:
    (A) Unconscious
    (B) Bleeding
    (C) Dehydrated
    (D) Immobilized

57. The fraction of the total radioactivity in the desired chemical form of a radiopharmaceutical is called:
    (A) Formulation strength
    (B) Radionuclide purity
    (C) Integrity of a formulation
    (D) Radiochemical purity

58. An arbitrary unit of X-ray attenuation used for Computerized Tomography (CT) scans is called:
    (A) Attenuation constant
    (B) Hounsfield unit
    (C) CT unit
    (D) Attenuation unit

59. Cs-137 source is certified to contain 150 μCi on January 2000. If the expected reading of Cs-137 on January 2010 is 119 μCi, and the actual reading is 110 μCi, what is the percent error of the dose calibrator?
    (A) 27%
    (B) 21%
    (C) 8%
    (D) 6%

60. Images obtained shortly after injection of white blood cells labeled with In-111 or Tc-99m are characterized by intense activity-up to 4 hr, but disappearing prior to 24 hr imaging-pulmonary activity. This phenomenon is caused by the fact that:
    (A) The mean driving pressure across the pulmonary circulation is higher than that in the systemic circulation
    (B) During the labeling procedure, neutrophils are deformed and became bigger
    (C) Activated neutrophils adhere to the pulmonary capillaries for a longer period than do nonactivated neutrophils
    (D) The pulmonary capillaries have an average diameter bigger than that of neutrophils

61. The distance that consists of the QRS complex, ST segment, and T wave is called:
    (A) QRT interval
    (B) QT interval
    (C) QT segment
    (D) QRT segment

62. Tc-99m-labeled leukocytes and Tc-99m sulfur colloid accumulate in the reticuloendothelial cells of the bone marrow. The distribution of marrow activity is similar for both radiopharmaceuticals with the exception of an acute or chronic bone infection. Osteomyelitis:
    (A) Stimulates uptake of leukocytes but suppresses uptake of sulfur colloid
    (B) Stimulates uptake of sulfur colloid but suppresses uptake of leukocytes
    (C) Stimulates uptake of leukocytes but does not affect uptake of sulfur colloid
    (D) Stimulates uptake of sulfur colloid but does not affect uptake of leukocytes

63. Continuous acquisition is an option to traditionally used step-and-shoot protocols and when it is used with proper reconstruction software the injection dose can be reduced by:
    (A) 0.1%
    (B) 1%
    (C) 5%
    (D) 50%

64. Attempts to localize the acute lower gastrointestinal bleeding involve colonoscopy, Tc-99m-labeled red blood cell scintigraphy, angiography, or a blend of these modalities. The sensitivity of each method of diagnosis is limited, with the most common cause of a negative study:
    (A) The hemorrhage cessation
    (B) The patient noncompliance
    (C) The patient selection
    (D) The technical difficulties

65. Flow images presented in Fig. 3.7 were obtained during gastrointestinal scintigraphy. Which two radiopharmaceuticals can be used in this type of procedure?
    (A) Tc-99-labeled red blood cells and Tc-99m sulfur colloid
    (B) Tc-99m mebrofenin and Tc-99m sulfur colloid
    (C) Tc-99-labeled white blood cells and Tc-99m mercaptoacetyltriglycine
    (D) Tc-99-labeled red blood cells and Tc-99-labeled white blood cells

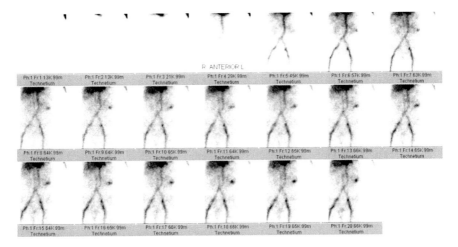

Fig. 3.7 Flow images during gastrointestinal scintigraphy

66. The use of new faster Computerized Tomography (CT) scanners for the evaluation of pulmonary embolism makes the diagnosis easier and as a result lesser than 5% of studies ordered for pulmonary embolism evaluation are ventilation–perfusion (V/Q) scans. CT studies when compared to V/Q scans:

    (A) Are more difficult to perform
    (B) Are less specific
    (C) Deliver higher effective dose to the patient
    (D) Have no contraindications

67. Free Tc-99mO$_4^-$ is an example of the radiochemical impurity in Tc-99m-tagged red blood cells (RBCs) preparation. During bleeding scan scintigraphy presence of free Tc-99m can be detected on:

    (A) Thyroid image
    (B) Liver image
    (C) Lung image
    (D) Brain image

68. The dual window subtraction technique is applied to:

    (A) Attenuation correction
    (B) Scatter correction
    (C) Resolution recovery
    (D) Linearity recovery

69. If the Tc-99m sulfur colloid calibrated activity is 6 mCi at 8:00 A.M., how much activity will be remaining 90 min later?
    (A) 5.0 mCi
    (B) 4.5 mCi
    (C) 4.0 mCi
    (D) 3.5 mCi

70. The morphine-augmented cholescintigraphy for the diagnosis of acute cholecystitis has high sensitivity and in clinical settings can be used as an alternative for:
    (A) Sincalide stimulation
    (B) Fatty meal stimulation
    (C) Delay imaging
    (D) Dynamic imaging

71. Chemically, the hormones produced in the adrenal cortex are:
    (A) Proteins
    (B) Sugars
    (C) Lipids
    (D) Catecholamines

72. According to the American Society of Nuclear Cardiology (ASNC) Imaging Guidelines, the radiopharmaceutical should be injected as close to peak exercise as possible. According to the guidelines after the radiotracer injection, patient should continue to exercise for at least:
    (A) 0.5–1.0 min
    (B) 1.0–1.5 min
    (C) 1.5–2 min
    (D) >2 min

73. A method employing two coincidence circuits with the standard and delayed time window is used for:
    (A) Attenuation correction
    (B) Scatter correction
    (C) Random events correction
    (D) Linearity recovery

74. The time from F-18 fluorodeoxyglucose (FDG) administration to the time of data acquisition has been shown to have a marked effect on FDG uptake. An increased interval between the injection and imaging uptake time will DECREASE radiotracer concentration in:
    (A) Tumor
    (B) Muscle
    (C) Bone marrow
    (D) Blood pool

75. Image presented in Fig. 3.8 was acquired during routine bone scintigraphy and
    it should be labeled with the following:

    (A) Plantar
    (B) Oblique
    (C) Posterior
    (D) Palmar

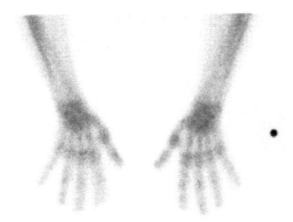

Fig. 3.8 Routine bone scintigraphy

76. More than a few of the main imaging modalities use ionizing radiation for
    cardiovascular diagnosis and/or treatment. Which of the following modalities
    is used for coronary artery plaque and calcification imaging?

    (A) Myocardial Perfusion Imaging (SPECT MPI)
    (B) Cardiac Positron Emission Tomography (PET)
    (C) Cardiac Computerized Tomography (CCT)
    (D) X-ray Fluoroscopy

77. The interaction of Al^{3+} with several Tc-99m radiopharmaceuticals is known to
    alter their biodistribution. Al^{3+} may react with Tc-99m methylene diphospho-
    nate (MDP) forming insoluble particles which:

    (A) Block the capillaries in lungs
    (B) Are taken up by the cells of reticuloendothelial system (RES) in liver and
        spleen
    (C) Are taken up by the cells of reticuloendothelial system (RES) in bone
        marrow
    (D) Block the arterioles in lungs

78. Open energy window is used when performing a wipe test and checking for surface contamination. Which of the following radionuclides CANNOT be detected on a wipe test?
    (A) Sm-153
    (B) Ga-67
    (C) Xe-133
    (D) Ga-68

79. The F-18 fluorodeoxyglucose (FDG) dose is calibrated for 22.7 mCi in 0.5 ml at 9:00 A.M. The patient arrives 35 min late for the scheduled positron emission tomography (PET) scan and the technologist wants to know how much activity will be remaining at 9:35 A.M.:
    (A) 18.2 mCi
    (B) 21.2 mCi
    (C) 31.2 mCi
    (D) 36.4 mCi

80. With the administration of oral contrast media for integrated Positron Emission Tomography/Computed Tomography (PET/CT) studies, CT-derived attenuation values are:
    (A) Overestimated
    (B) Underestimated
    (C) Not applicable
    (D) Not performed

81. Which of the following symptoms/conditions can indicate the presence of gastrointestinal bleeding?
    (A) Hematopoiesis
    (B) Melena
    (C) Subdural hematoma
    (D) Intermittent hematuria

82. Diagnostic strategies for the management of patients with suspected pulmonary embolism (PE) should include pretest clinical probability, D-dimer assays, and imaging tests. D-dimer helps diagnose or rule out all of the following thrombotic diseases and conditions EXCEPT:
    (A) Pulmonary embolism (PE)
    (B) Deep venous thrombosis (DVT)
    (C) Disseminated intravascular coagulation (DIC)
    (D) Urinary tract infection (UTI)

83. A sodium-iodide (NaI) crystal activated with thallium is the most widely used type of solid scintillation detectors. Activation with thallium:

(A) Produces centers of luminescence
(B) Prolongs crystal longevity
(C) Prevents crystal deformation
(D) Stabilizes crystal structure

84. The appearance of the "Reverse redistribution" phenomenon, the presence of a focal defect in rest images that was not seen on stress images, or presence of a focal defect in stress images that appears more severe on rest images, can be created by all of the following EXCEPT:

(A) Tissue attenuation on the rest images caused by position shift
(B) Motion artifact on the rest images
(C) Dose extravasation
(D) Misalignment on SPECT slices

85. Figure 3.9 images were acquired during routine bone scintigraphy after intravenous 26.6 mCi of Tc-99m methylene diphsophonate (MDP) administration. Which of the following statements is most consistent with the finding from the scan?

(A) Normal scan
(B) Rib fractures
(C) Bone metastases
(D) Paget's disease

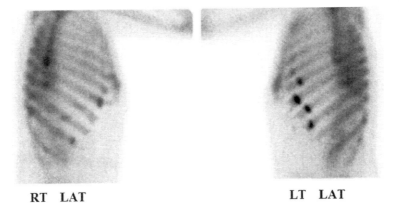

RT   LAT   **LT   LAT**

Fig. 3.9 Routine bone scintigraphy

86. Which of the following preventive measures/devices should be used in rooms where radioactive gases are used?
    (A) Negative air pressure
    (B) Breathing masks
    (C) High efficiency particulate air (HEPA) filters
    (D) Air locks

87. The chemical purity of the radiopharmaceutical is the fraction of the material in the desired chemical form. Chemical impurities:
    (A) Arise from the breakdown of the material
    (B) Are buffers
    (C) Are additives
    (D) All of the above are impurities

88. Scatter fraction is defined as the fraction of the total counts that are from scatter and is related to all of the following EXCEPT:
    (A) Energy window width
    (B) Acquisition time
    (C) Energy resolution
    (D) Photon energy

89. A 6.0 mCi In-111 Pentetreotide dose calibrated for Monday 8:00 A.M. was ordered from the radiopharmacy. Unfortunately the patient was not able to keep the appointment and the dose was never used. How much activity was remaining on Wednesday of the same week at 10:00 A.M.? (Decay factor is 0.600)
    (A) 4.4 mCi
    (B) 3.6 mCi
    (C) 2.4 mCi
    (D) 2.0 mCi

90. The most dependable method for detecting the extent, direction, and frequency of cardiac motion during myocardial perfusion imaging is:
    (A) Inspecting the cardiac sinogram
    (B) Inspecting the rotating planar images
    (C) Inspecting a summed planar frames image
    (D) Observing the patient during acquisition

91. The transverse colon is the part of the colon that extends from:
    (A) The cecum to the hepatic flexure
    (B) The hepatic flexure to the splenic flexure
    (C) The splenic flexure to the beginning of the sigmoid colon
    (D) The descending colon to the rectum

92. The most favorable separation of right and left ventricles on Equilibrium Radionuclide Angiography (ERNA) is generally achieved in the left anterior obliquity at a 45-degree angle. The left anterior oblique (LAO) examination presents views of the cardiac:

    (A) Anterior and apical segments
    (B) Inferior wall and posterobasal segments
    (C) Septal, inferoapical, and lateral walls
    (D) Septal and anterior walls

93. Simultaneous absorption of two or more gamma rays in the gamma camera crystal is called:

    (A) Pulse pileup
    (B) Scatter
    (C) Sum peaks
    (D) Attenuation

94. When short cardiac beats of gated cardiac scintigraphy do not contribute counts to the later gating intervals, the produced phenomenon on SPECT images viewed in cinematic mode is called:

    (A) Flickering
    (B) Skipping
    (C) Count add-on
    (D) Limping

95. The display on the Fig. 3.10 presents reconstruction reoriented SPECT data to the patient's heart and created:

    (A) Short axis slices
    (B) Vertical long axis slices
    (C) Long axis slices
    (D) Horizontal long axis

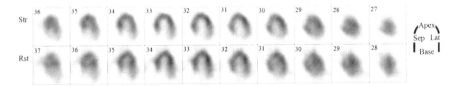

Fig. 3.10 Reconstruction reoriented SPECT data

96. People who inhale tobacco smoke are exposed to higher concentrations of radioactivity than nonsmokers. Radioactive carcinogens in tobacco emit:
    (A) Alpha particles
    (B) Beta particles
    (C) Gamma ray
    (D) X-ray

97. The distance that the positron passes from its origin to the point of the annihilation is called positron range. Which of the following radionuclides has the highest maximum positron range?
    (A) Carbon-11
    (B) Fluor-18
    (C) Rubidium-82
    (D) Nitrogen-13

98. A three-dimensional representation of the signal measured at a given angle in the imaging plane at varying distances along the detector array is called:
    (A) Linogram
    (B) Sinogram
    (C) 3 DM (three-dimensional)
    (D) Cryptogram

99. 5 mCi Tc-99m of mebrofenin is needed for a hepatobiliary scan at 5:00 P.M. If the unit dose was being prepared by radiopharmacy at 10:00 A.M. same day, how much activity with the dose contain?
    (A) 22.2 mCi
    (B) 15.10 mCi
    (C) 11.2 mCi
    (D) 7.2 mCi

100. The relationship between coronary blood flow and the myocardial uptake of radiotracers is not linear, and all commonly used radiopharmaceuticals show a plateau at higher blood flow levels. This property of radiotracers is called:
    (A) Saturation
    (B) Roll-off
    (C) Flow reserve
    (D) Limitation

101. Coronary artery disease is an immune inflammatory process, which, over decades, results in arterial narrowing. All of the following factors can quicken this process EXCEPT:
    (A) Homocysteine
    (B) Increased high-density lipoprotein (HDL) cholesterol
    (C) Increased levels of low-density lipoprotein (LDL) cholesterol
    (D) Lipoprotein

102. Partial volume effect observed with tomographic myocardial perfusion imaging may make it difficult to visualize the left ventricle (LV) cavity of patients with small hearts, and will lead to the overestimation of the left ventricle ejection fraction (LVEF). Overestimation of the LVEF is caused by:
    (A) Underestimation of the end systolic (ES) volume
    (B) Underestimation of the end diastolic (ED) volume
    (C) Overestimation of the end systolic (ES) volume
    (D) Overestimation of the end diastolic (ED) volume

103. When performing a daily intrinsic flood, the activity of a point source of Tc-99m should be adjusted to generate a measured counting rate of no greater than 25,000 cps to prevent:
    (A) Camera overheating
    (B) Dead-time counting losses
    (C) Photomultiplier tubes (PM) stunning
    (D) Fuse melting

104. The 17-segment semiquantitative visual scores have been shown to provide important prognostic information. The maximal, no heart visualized abnormal summed stress score (SSS) is equal to:
    (A) 85
    (B) 68
    (C) 51
    (D) 34

105. Figure 3.11. A 64-year-old man presented with abdominal pain. Computerized Tomography (CT) revealed rim-enhancing hepatic lesions and the patient was referred to the nuclear medicine department for further evaluation. The patient was injected with 6.1 mCi of In-111 Octreoscan and images were acquired 4 h later. Findings of the scan are most consistent with the clinical diagnosis of:
    (A) Liver hemangioma
    (B) Liver cyst
    (C) Carcinoid tumor
    (D) Hepatitis C

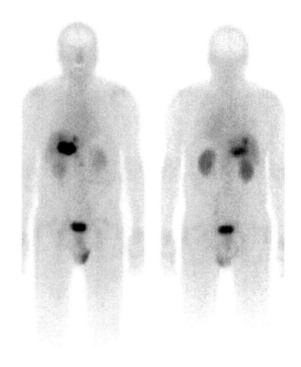

RT   ANT   LT   LT   POST   RT

Fig. 3.11 In-111 Octreoscan scintigraphy

106. If radiation interacts with the atoms of the deoxyribonucleic acid (DNA) molecule, or some other cellular component critical to the survival of the cell, it is referred to as:
    (A) Ionization effect of radiation
    (B) Excitation effect of radiation
    (C) Direct effect of radiation
    (D) Indirect effect of radiation

107. In the photoelectric effect, an electron is ejected from its orbit with the kinetic energy the same as the energy of the gamma ray which hit it minus:
    (A) Repulsive force
    (B) Binding energy
    (C) Attractive force
    (D) Gamma ray coefficient

108. Spatial resolution and spatial linearity of gamma camera should be checked with the four-quadrant bar phantom at least weekly, with a five- to ten-million-count transmission image obtained. The lead bars should be visually resolvable in:

(A) At least three quadrants
(B) At least two quadrants
(C) At least one quadrant
(D) All quadrants

109. A Tc-99m methylene diphosphonate (MDP) kit is being prepared at 7:00 A.M. for a scheduled skeletal scintigraphy. If 25 mCi doses are needed at 8:00, 10:00, and 1:00 P.M., what is the minimum activity that should be placed in the vial at 7:00 A.M. to accommodate scheduled procedures?

(A) 53 mCi
(B) 63 mCi
(C) 84 mCi
(D) 113 mCi

110. The sensitivity of the exercise SPECT myocardial perfusion imaging for recognizing disease in individual coronary arteries is the highest in:

(A) Left Anterior Descending (LAD)
(B) Right coronary artery (RCA)
(C) Left circumflex artery (LCX)
(D) Triple vessel disease (LAD, RCA, LCX)

111. The portion of the abdomen and pelvis which lies within the peritoneum is called the intraperitoneal space. Which the following organ(s) is/are situated intraperitoneally?

(A) Kidneys
(B) Pancreas
(C) Liver
(D) Bladder

112. The most common adverse reaction with pharmacologic stress agents dipyridamole and dobutamine is:

(A) Dyspnea
(B) Palpitation
(C) Chest pain
(D) Headache

113. Ionization chambers, proportional counters, and Geiger–Mueller survey meters are examples of what type radiation detectors?

(A) Scintillation counters
(B) Gas-filled radiation detectors
(C) Water-based radiation detectors
(D) Coincidence detectors

114. Tc-99m mercaptoacetyltriglycine is the most commonly used radiopharmaceutical for:
    (A) Adrenal scintigraphy
    (B) Renal scintigraphy
    (C) Neuroendocrine tumor imaging
    (D) V-P shunt patency imaging

115. The Fig. 3.12 displays four different I-123 thyroid scans images where image "A" demonstrates a normal thyroid gland. Image "C" findings are more consistent with the clinical diagnoses of:
    (A) Hypothyroidism
    (B) Grave's disease
    (C) Multinodular goiter
    (D) Autonomously hyperfunctioning thyroid nodule

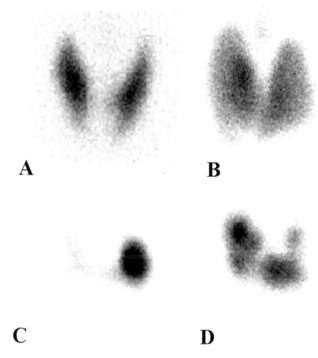

Fig. 3.12 I-123 thyroid scans images

116. For pregnant workers, a fetal monitor may be issued to track the dose and ensure that the fetus does not receive a dose in excess of:
    (A) 50 mrem/month
    (B) 500 mrem/month
    (C) 1,000 mrem per gestational period
    (D) 1,000 mrem/year

117. The process when an electron moves from a ground state to an excited state or from a lower energy state to a higher energy state is called:

(A) Transition
(B) Transformation
(C) Ionization
(D) Excitation

118. A low-pass filter (e.g., Hanning or Butterworth) eliminates:

(A) Spatial frequencies above a cutoff frequency
(B) Spatial frequencies below a cutoff frequency
(C) Spatial frequencies above and below a cutoff frequency
(D) Accidently detected spatial frequencies

119. The MAG3 package insert recommends minimum volume of 4 ml for kit reconstitution. If 90 mCi mercaptoacetyltriglycine kit is prepared from a vial of bulk Tc-99m that has concentration of 68 mCi/ml, what volume of saline is needed to be added to meet the minimum recommended total volume of 4 ml?

(A) 0.7 ml
(B) 1.7 ml
(C) 2.7 ml
(D) 3.7 ml

120. Metastatic tumor, cyst, infarction, hematoma, trauma etc. will appear on Tc-99m sulfur colloid liver spleen scintigraphy as:

(A) Hot spot
(B) Cold spot
(C) Patchy area
(D) Ring sign

121. The arterial Circle of Willis, also called Willis' Circle, is a circle of arteries that supply blood to:

(A) The liver
(B) The spleen
(C) The brain
(D) The uterus

122. A catecholamine/metabolites secreting embryonic tumor of the peripheral sympathetic nervous system is called:

(A) Neuroblastoma
(B) Germ cell tumor
(C) Wilm's tumor
(D) Adrenocortical tumor

123. The blank scan is performed daily on Positron Emission Tomography (PET) scanners using a Ge-68 transmission source. The term blank scan reflects:
    (A) The absence of any material in the field of view (FOV)
    (B) The absence of emission data
    (C) The absence of patient
    (D) The absence of technologist

124. The most common type of lymphoma that occurs in the USA and Western Europe is derived from:
    (A) B cells
    (B) T cells
    (C) Mantle cells
    (D) Plasma cells

125. The myocardial perfusion can be estimated by analyzing the stress images-labeled A with the rest images-labeled B. Images presented on the Fig. 3.13 and displayed as a bull's eye polar plot indicate presence of:
    (A) Irreversible defect
    (B) Reversible defect
    (C) Wall motion abnormalities
    (D) Apical thinning

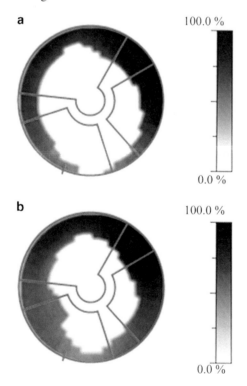

Fig. 3.13 Bull's eye polar plot

126. Which of the following standard myocardial perfusion protocols deliver the highest effective dose to the patient?

(A) Tc-99m Sestamibi 2 day protocol
(B) Dual isotope Tl-201 and Tc-99m sestamibi same day protocol
(C) Tl-201 stress-reinjection protocol
(D) F-18 fluorodeoxyglucose protocol

127. Photons are a form of electromagnetic radiation and are characterized by all of the following EXCEPT:

(A) Photon mass is equal to electron mass
(B) Photons have zero charge
(C) Photons velocity is that of the speed of light
(D) Photons are more penetrating than charged particles of similar energy

128. A surgically implanted tube that connects the peritoneal cavity and the superior vena cava to drain accumulated fluid from the peritoneal cavity is known as:

(A) Ventriculo-Peritoneal shunt
(B) LeVeen shunt
(C) Left to right shunt
(D) Hemodialysis shunt

129. A 14 year old child who weighs 125 pound is referred for renal scintigraphy with Tc-99m mercaptoacetyltriglycine (MAG3). If the adult dose is 9 mCi, what is the pediatric dose for that child according to Clark's formula?

(A) 10.5 mCi
(B) 9.5 mCi
(C) 8.5 mCi
(D) 7.5 mCi

130. An ultimate treatment for patients who are nonresponsive to or cannot tolerate other available therapies for a particular illness and whose prognosis is often poor is called:

(A) Standard therapy
(B) Retreatment
(C) Salvage therapy
(D) Consolidation therapy

131. An organ that removes old red blood cells, holds a reserve of blood in case of hemorrhagic shock, and synthesizes antibodies in its white pulp is called:

(A) The spleen
(B) Bone marrow
(C) The thymus
(D) The liver

132. All generic names for monoclonal antibodies end with the suffix "mab" and antibodies directed against tumor antigens often include the syllable "tu." General name "tuximab" describes:
(A) A chimeric monoclonal antibody to a tumor antigen
(B) The humanized monoclonal antibody to a tumor antigen
(C) A mouse monoclonal antibody to a tumor antigen
(D) A cloned monoclonal antibody to a tumor antigen

133. A quality control procedure performed by comparing the extrinsic and intrinsic uniformity floods is called:
(A) Spatial resolution
(B) Collimator integrity
(C) Spatial uniformity
(D) Collimator linearity

134. In-111 ibritumomab, a component of Zevalin regimen is administered for what purpose?
(A) To saturate CD-20 epitope of B cells in the circulation and in the spleen
(B) To confirm normal biodistribution of the labeled antibody
(C) To determine the therapeutic dose of Zevalin
(D) To ensure proper antibody-epitope binding

135. Figure 3.14 presents the schematic diagram of a hepatobiliary tract. What part of the hepatobiliary tree represents label "d"?
(A) Sphincter of Oddi
(B) Cystic duct
(C) Common bile duct
(D) Common hepatic duct

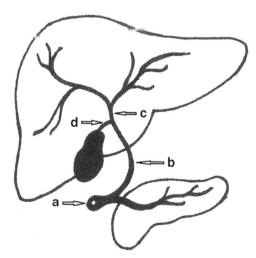

Fig. 3.14 Schematic diagram of the hepatobiliary tract (*Illustration by Sabina Moniuszko*)

136. According to the American Society of Nuclear Cardiology (ASNC) "Recommendations for reducing radiation exposure in myocardial perfusion imaging," widening the energy window and count consistency methods:
    (A) Require immediate implementation
    (B) Require further validation
    (C) Are not useful
    (D) Offer some advantages when imaging larger patients

137. Comparatively greater concentration of Tc-99m methylene diphosphonate (MDP) in the effusion rather than in other soft-tissues at the typical time of imaging, results from all of the following EXCEPT:
    (A) Slow back-diffusion
    (B) Large distribution volume
    (C) Excessive capillary permeability
    (D) Drug interaction

138. Increasing the thickness of inorganic scintillation detector will result in the detector:
    (A) Higher resolution and lower sensitivity
    (B) Higher resolution and higher resolution
    (C) Lower resolution and higher sensitivity
    (D) Lower resolution and lower sensitivity

139. If a vial of generator elute contains 630 mCi Tc-99m and 43 μCi of Mo-99, what is the Molybdenum to Technetium concentration?
    (A) 0.15 μCi Mo-99/mCi Tc-99m
    (B) 0.13 μCi Mo-99/mCi Tc-99m
    (C) 0.07 μCi Mo-99/mCi Tc-99m
    (D) 0.03 μCi Mo-99/mCi Tc-99m

140. To lessen the ability for the development of human anti-mouse antibodies (HAMA), it is possible to retain the immunospecific portion of the antibody that has been encoded as a murine protein, while replacing a large portion of the remainder of the mouse immunoglobulin g (IgG) molecule with:
    (A) A monkey Immunoglobulin G sequence
    (B) A smaller portion of a mouse Immunoglobulin G
    (C) A large portion of mouse Immunoglobulin M
    (D) A human Immunoglobulin G sequence

141. There are normally 33 vertebrae in humans: how many of them are located in thoracic region?
    (A) 5
    (B) 7
    (C) 9
    (D) 12

142. Before scheduling treatment with Zevalin, all of the following lab data should be available to confirm that the patients meet the eligibility criteria EXCEPT:
(A) Recent (within 1–2 weeks) complete blood count with attention to absolute neutrophils and platelets count
(B) Recent (within 6–8 weeks) bone marrow biopsy results to confirm less than 25% involvement.
(C) Recent (within 1–2 weeks) liver function tests
(D) Initial biopsy confirmation of CD20 expression

143. Star-shaped activity seen on images at the site of injection that could possibly impair visualization of nearby structures is caused by the phenomenon known as:
(A) Septal penetration
(B) Defective collimator
(C) Overheated photomultiplier (PM) tube
(D) Detector non-uniformity

144. According to the sulfur colloid package extended beyond the recommended heating time will result in colloidal particles that are:
(A) Crystallized
(B) Dispersed
(C) Too little
(D) Too large

145. Curves of cortical kidney activity are displayed in Fig. 3.15. Graph "a" presents a normal pattern with a prompt increase in activity and spontaneous washout. Curve of cortical kidney activity displayed on graph "b" is described as:
(A) Dilated nonobstructed pattern
(B) Blunted response pattern
(C) Obstructed pattern
(D) Golden pattern

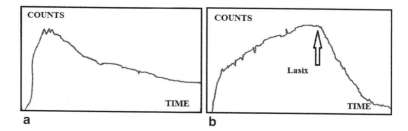

Fig. 3.15 Curves of cortical kidney activity (*Illustration by Sabina Moniuszko*)

146. By federal law all diagnostic doses must be within 20% of the prescribed dose. A deviation of more than 10% but less than 20% of administered therapeutic dose constitutes:
    (A) Acceptable event
    (B) Recordable event
    (C) Reportable event
    (D) Misadministration

147. There are four elementary radioactive decay processes. Inverse beta decay is also known as:
    (A) Beta minus decay
    (B) Alpha decay
    (C) Electron capture
    (D) Beta positive decay (positron decay)

148. The pinhole collimator provides the best resolution for small organs positioned a short distance from the aperture. Increasing the distance will result in all of the following EXCEPT:
    (A) Decreased sensitivity
    (B) Decreased resolution
    (C) Decreased count rate
    (D) Increased the apparent size of the object

149. A vial of generator elute contains 450 mCi Tc-99m and 51 µCi of Mo-99. This vial will expire in:
    (A) 287 min
    (B) 247 min
    (C) 3.7 h
    (D) 2.7 h

150. Any lymph node that receives lymph drainage directly from the tumor site is called:
    (A) The local lymph node
    (B) The metastatic lymph node
    (C) The regional lymph node
    (D) The sentinel node

151. Treatment of hyperthyroidism with antithyroid medications must be given for 6 months to 2 years, in order to be effective. The two main antithyroid drugs are:
    (A) Methimazole and Propylthiouracil
    (B) Methimazole and Propranolol
    (C) Metronidazole and Propylthiouracil
    (D) Metronidazole and Propranolol

152. Which of the following is the imaging agent of choice for lung perfusion scintigraphy?
    (A) Radiolabeled macroaggregated bovine albumin
    (B) Radiolabeled diethylenetriamine pentaacetic acid
    (C) Radiolabeled hexamethylpropyleneamine oxime
    (D) Radiolabeled macroaggregated human albumin

153. The basic procedure in filtered backprojection reconstruction technique converting the spatial domain into the frequency space is known as:
    (A) Filtering
    (B) Volume rendering
    (C) Fourier transform
    (D) Convoluting

154. The normal thyroid gland images should have smooth contour and homogenous tracer localization. Relatively less activity present at the periphery of the lobes:
    (A) Is a normal variation
    (B) Is an artifact
    (C) Indicates thyroid pathology
    (D) Requires additional testing

155. A 42 year old woman with right upper quadrant abdominal pain was referred for hepatobiliary scintigraphy and acquired images are shown in Fig. 3.16. What type of liver cells are responsible for uptake of Tc-99m mebrofenin?
    (A) Kupffer cells
    (B) Hepatocytes
    (C) Hepatic sinusoidal endothelial cells
    (D) Hepatic stellate cells

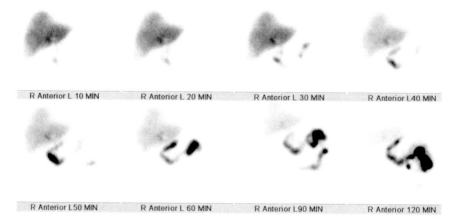

Fig. 3.16 Hepatobiliary scintigraphy

156. The effects of radiation usually associated with exposures to low levels of radiation exposure over a long period of time are known as:
    (A) Stochastic effects
    (B) Chronic effects
    (C) Deterministic effects
    (D) Side effects

157. The photoelectric effect is most likely to happen in:
    (A) Water
    (B) Pb collimator
    (C) The human body
    (D) Air

158. Which of the following statements describing the thyroid probe (TP) counter is TRUE?
    (A) Counting efficiency of the TP increases with the distance between the source and the detector
    (B) Counting efficiency of the TP does not change with the distance between the source and the detector
    (C) TP requires a lead collimator
    (D) TP does not need calibration

159. If a radioactive source is producing 24,506 counts per minute (cpm), what is the acceptable range of values at 95% confidence level?
    (A) Between 24,193 and 24,819 cpm
    (B) Between 24,411 and 24,801 cpm
    (C) Between 24,606 and 24,788 cpm
    (D) Between 24,831 and 24,681 cpm

160. A "hot" nodule present on an I-123 thyroid scan is almost always benign and repeatedly characterizes a hyperfunctioning adenoma. The probability of the nodule toxicity:
    (A) Decreases with time
    (B) Increases with the nodule size
    (C) Decreases with the nodule size
    (D) Increases with time

161. A normal hematocrit is approximately what percentage of a given blood volume?
    (A) 25%
    (B) 35%
    (C) 45%
    (D) 55%

162. According to the Society of Nuclear Medicine "SNM Procedure Guideline for Therapy of Thyroid Disease with I-131 (Sodium Iodide)," typically administered activity for treatment of presumed thyroid cancer in the neck or mediastinal lymph nodes is in the range:
    (A) 50–100 mCi
    (B) 100–150 mCi
    (C) 150–200 mCi
    (D) 200–250 mCi

163. Geometric efficiency of scintillation detector is the highest when used in the:
    (A) Gamma camera equipped with pinhole collimator
    (B) Well counter
    (C) Thyroid probe
    (D) Dual-head gamma camera

164. The Patlak plot, the modified Brenner and the area-under-the curve (AUC) methods are techniques of:
    (A) Quantitative measurements of bone remodeling
    (B) Quantitative measurements of gallbladder function
    (C) Quantitative measurements of renal function
    (D) Quantitative measurements of lung perfusion

165. What part of urinary tract is indicated by the arrow in Fig. 3.17?
    (A) Right renal pelvis
    (B) Left renal pelvis
    (C) Left renal pyramid
    (D) Right renal pyramid

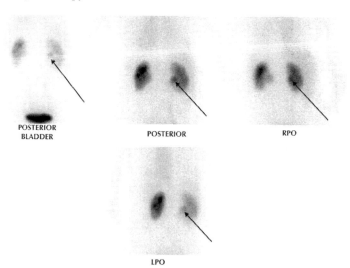

Fig. 3.17 MAG3 renal scintigraphy-static images

166. All of the following organizations are entitled to develop rules governing transport of radioactive materials EXCEPT:
    (A) Department of Transportation (DOT)
    (B) Department of Energy (DOE)
    (C) FedEx
    (D) Postal Service

167. What biologically significant constituent does gallium most closely resemble?
    (A) Potassium
    (B) Thallium
    (C) Indium
    (D) Iron

168. All of the following parameters of the uptake probe should be set when thyroid function measurements are performed EXCEPT:
    (A) High voltage settings
    (B) Photopeak settings
    (C) Energy window
    (D) Dead time settings

169. If a radioactive source produces the exposure of 80 mR/h at the distance of 3 ft, how far away should the technologist stand to reduce the exposure rate to 5 mR/h?
    (A) 6 ft
    (B) 8 ft
    (C) 10 ft
    (D) 12 ft

170. The two most frequently affected sites in Paget's disease are the bones:
    (A) Skull and tibia
    (B) Femur and cervical spine
    (C) Pelvis and lumbar spine
    (D) Thoracic spine and humerus

171. An ultimate treatment for patients who are nonresponsive to or cannot tolerate other available therapies for a particular illness and whose prognosis is often poor is called:
    (A) Standard therapy
    (B) Retreatment
    (C) Salvage therapy
    (D) Consolidation therapy

172. The most prevalent modes of myocardial perfusion (MPI) tomographic acquisition is the "step-and-shoot" and "continuous technique." Small amount of blurring is present if the images are acquired by:

    (A) Step and shoot
    (B) Both methods
    (C) Continuous
    (D) Neither method

173. A dose calibrator is used in nuclear medicine departments to measure the radioactivity of radionuclide samples. In the process of measurement:

    (A) The number of ionizations is converted to curie (Ci) or becquerel (Bq)
    (B) The number of cts is converted to curie (Ci) or becquerel (Bq)
    (C) The number of ionizations is converted to rad or gray (Gy)
    (D) The number of cts is converted to rem or sievert (Sv)

174. I-123 metaiodobenzylguanidine (MIBG), an analog of guanidine that shares the same neuronal transport and storage mechanisms with norepinephrine, has been used to evaluate:

    (A) The sympathetic activity
    (B) The parasympathetic activity
    (C) The autonomous activity
    (D) The central brain activity

175. Figure 3.18 displays thyroid images acquired 6 h after I-123 oral administration. Findings of presented thyroid scintigraphy – arrows – are most consistent with the presence of:

    (A) Cold nodule
    (B) Hot nodule
    (C) Defective collimator
    (D) Motion defect

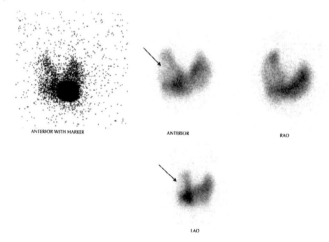

Fig. 3.18 Thyroid images acquired 6 hrs after I-123 oral administration

176. Nuclear Medicine wastes fall in the low-level waste class and can be grouped in one of the following categories EXCEPT:

    (A) Radioactive gases
    (B) Liquid wastes
    (C) Jelly wastes
    (D) Solid wastes

177. All of the following are examples of cyclotron-produced radionuclides EXCEPT:

    (A) F-18
    (B) Tl-201
    (C) I-123
    (D) I-131

178. Intraoperative probes are broadly used devices in the surgical management of cancer. They are most commonly utilized to localize:

    (A) Metastatic lung carcinoma
    (B) Sentinel node
    (C) Radiolabeled antibody
    (D) Shunt obstruction

179. A radioactive source produces the exposure of 25 mR/h with 2HVL in place. What would be the new exposure rate with two half-value layers added?

    (A) 6.3 mR/h
    (B) 7.4 mR/h
    (C) 8.2 mR/h
    (D) 9.1 mR/h

180. All of the following diagnostic methods can be used for the identification of hibernating myocardium EXCEPT:

    (A) FDG PET
    (B) SPECT MPI
    (C) Dobutamine echocardiography
    (D) Stress electrocardiography

181. Coronary blood flow to the left ventricle occurs predominantly in:

    (A) Left ventricle diastole
    (B) Left ventricle systole
    (C) Left atrium diastole
    (D) Left atrium systole

182. Esmolol, cardioselective beta-receptor blocker, is used for the lessening of the severe side effects of which pharmacological stress agent?
    (A) Adenosine
    (B) Dipyridamole
    (C) Dobutamine
    (D) Regadenosan

183. Each quality test (QC) performed in the nuclear medicine department must be documented. All of the following data should be included in this description EXCEPT:
    (A) The date and the time of the test
    (B) The initials/signature of technologist performing the test
    (C) The signature of lead technologist
    (D) The make, model, and serial number of any reference source used

184. Which of the following radioisotopes approved in the USA for use in the treatment of bone metastases has a significant gamma emission and can be used both for imaging and therapy?
    (A) Sr-89
    (B) P-32
    (C) Ra-223
    (D) Sm-153

185. What views were the lung perfusion images in Fig 3.19 acquired?
    (A) Anterior and posterior
    (B) Right lateral and left lateral
    (C) Right posterior oblique and left posterior oblique
    (D) Right anterior oblique and left posterior oblique

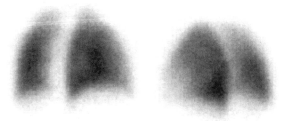

Fig. 3.19 Lung perfusion images

186. Thermoluminescent dosimeter (TLD) badges enclose thermoluminescence material and are acceptable whole-body and hand dose monitoring methods. Thermoluminescence substance:

   (A) Emits light after heating
   (B) Emits heat after lightning
   (C) Produces electric charge after heating
   (D) Produces light when electric current apply

187. Beta particles are subatomic particles ejected from the nucleus of some radio-active atoms. Beta particles:

   (A) Are bigger than alpha particles
   (B) Are positively or negatively charged electrons
   (C) Can be stopped by a single sheet of paper
   (D) Originate outside of the atomic nucleus

188. Gamma cameras are calibrated to ensure a high degree of uniformity. Correction tables for changes in camera sensitivity over time are derived from:

   (A) Daily floods
   (B) Weekly bars
   (C) Monthly high-count floods
   (D) All of the above

189. Thin layer chromatography counts for the evaluated dimercaptosuccinic acid (DMSA) kit are as follows:

   - free Tc-99m at the solvent front: 3,842 counts per minute (cpm),
   - Tc99m DMSA at the origin: 99,897 counts per minute (cpm)
   - background: 391 counts per minute (cpm)

   What is the purity of the DMSA kit?

   (A) 97%
   (B) 96%
   (C) 95%
   (D) 94%

190. Myocardial perfusion stress data, displayed in the form of polar image, is generated when the patient's stress perfusion plot is matched with:

   (A) Patient's rest perfusion plot
   (B) Data base abnormal study of an age and gender matched population
   (C) Data base normal study of an age and gender matched population
   (D) Previously performed stress perfusion data

191. Substance that inhibits thyroid hormone synthesis, leading to increased thyroid-stimulating hormone (TSH) production and resulting in an enlargement of the thyroid is called:
    (A) Immunogene
    (B) Goitrogen
    (C) Allergen
    (D) Carcinogen

192. The normal value of lung/heart ratio on scans utilizing Tc-99m sestamibi is:
    (A) >1.0
    (B) >0.44
    (C) <0.44
    (D) <1.0

193. When using a Co-57 sheet source for extrinsic quality assurance of camera uniformity, there may be visible contamination from higher energy gamma rays arising from other isotopes, namely:
    (A) Co-56 and Co-58
    (B) Co-59 and Co-60
    (C) Co-50 and Co-73
    (D) Co-51 and Co-52

194. Which of the following statements correctly describes transient ischemic dilation (TID) as a quantitative marker of myocardial perfusion imaging (MPI) SPECT?
    (A) Abnormal TID values correspond to stress-induced RV dysfunction
    (B) Normal TID values exclude severe coronary artery disease (CAD)
    (C) Cutoff values for an abnormal TID ratio vary
    (D) Higher TID ratio suggests a lesser ischemic burden

195. Presented images were obtained during routine sentinel node scintigraphy performed in woman with a biopsy-proven carcinoma of the breast after intradermal, peritumoral injections of Tc-99m sulfur colloid. The body contour seen on the images was obtained with:
    (A) Internal transmission source
    (B) Manual tracing with external source
    (C) External transmission source
    (D) Automatic tracing with external source

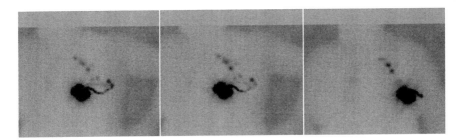

Fig. 3.20 Routine sentinel node scintigraphy

196. Which of the following radiopharmaceuticals will deliver the highest, rad/mCi whole body dose?
    (A) Tl-201 chloride
    (B) Ga-67 citrate
    (C) F-18 fluorodeoxyglucose
    (D) Tc-99m sestamibi

197. Molybdenum-99 and Technetium-99 are:
    (A) Isotones
    (B) Isobars
    (C) Isomers
    (D) Isotopes

198. The intrinsic resolution of the gamma camera is influenced by all of the system components EXCEPT:
    (A) Pulse height analyzer
    (B) Collimator
    (C) Crystal
    (D) Photomultiplier tubes (PMTs)

199. A gastric emptying study was performed with Tc-99m sulfur colloid mixed with oatmeal. Counts were derived from a Region of Interest (ROI) drawn over the images obtained immediately and 1-h post consumption of radioactive meal and are listed below:
    – immediate image: 75,340 cts anterior view and 73,245 cts posterior view
    – 1-h postconsumption image: 50,345 anterior view and 48,135 posterior view

    What is the percentage of gastric emptying at 60 min?
    (A) 26%
    (B) 43%
    (C) 49%
    (D) 52%

200. 16-frame gating left ventricle ejection fraction (LVEF) measurements show 4% increase in ejection fraction when compared to 8-frame gating. 16-frame gating LVEF estimations are higher because:

    (A) 16-frame gating localizes end diastole frame more precisely
    (B) 16-frame gating localizes end systole frame more precisely
    (C) 8-frame gating localizes end diastole frame more precisely
    (D) 8-frame gating localizes end systole frame more precisely

201. The American Heart Association uses four links in the Chain of Survival to illustrate the important time-sensitive actions for victims of Ventricular Fibrillation Sudden Cardiac Arrest (VF SCA). The second link in this chain is described as:

    (A) Early delivery of a shock with defibrillator
    (B) Early recognition of the emergency
    (C) Early bystander CPR
    (D) Early advanced life support

202. Blood flow images obtained during triple phase bone scintigraphy reflect:

    (A) Osteoblastic reaction to the primary disease
    (B) Degree of soft tissue involvement
    (C) Osteoblastic reaction to the primary disease
    (D) Vascularity of involved tissue

203. Decreasing the filter cutoff will provide very smooth images in addition to:

    (A) Loss of detail
    (B) Amplified noise
    (C) Increased resolution
    (D) Increased background

204. The pelvis can be difficult to evaluate when there is overlying bladder activity. In patients with pelvic symptoms, all of the following may be helpful in visualization of pelvic bony structures EXCEPT:

    (A) Repeating images after voiding
    (B) Masking technique
    (C) Sitting-on-detector view
    (D) Lateral views

205. An 85 years old woman with anemia secondary to acute blood loss underwent recent angiographic procedure utilizing a right groin approach. Presented images were acquired after 18.9 mCi of Tc-99m-labeled RBC's. Images demonstrate progressive radionuclide accumulation and are most consistent with the presence of:

    (A) Active bleeding in the transverse colon
    (B) Abdominal wall hematoma
    (C) Hematoma of the thigh
    (D) Active sigmoidal bleeding

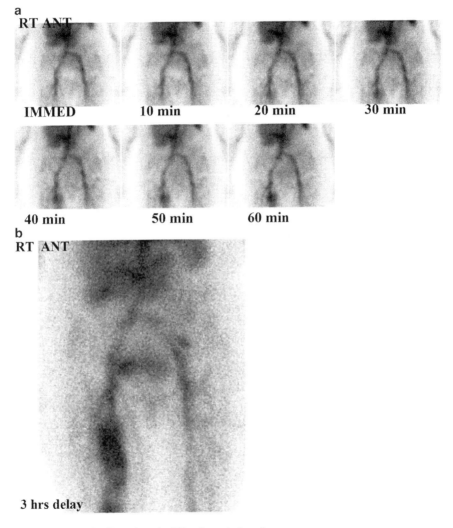

Fig. 3.21 (a) & (b) Gastrointestinal bleeding scintigraphy

206. Which of the following is the critical organ for Tc-99m methylene diphospho-
    nate (MDP) bone scintigraphy?
    (A) Gallbladder
    (B) Kidney
    (C) Bladder
    (D) Liver

207. Which of the following radiopharmaceuticals is best suited for performing
    renal function studies?
    (A) Tc-99m MAG3
    (B) I-131 Hippuran
    (C) Tc-99m DMSA
    (D) Tc-99m DTPA

208. Which of the following methods is most commonly used in nuclear pharmacy
    for determining alumina contamination?
    (A) Colorimetric test
    (B) Hemacytometer determination
    (C) Millipore filtration
    (D) Spectrum analysis

209. A radioactive source in 20 ml of volume is reading 6.4 mCi during the dose
    calibrator geometry test. What is the percent error caused by volume change
    if the reference source in 6 ml of volume is reading 6.9 mCi?
    (A) −7%
    (B) −6%
    (C) 6%
    (D) 7%

210. The composite image of the right ventricle (RV) in first pass studies includes
    all the frames between the first frame, in which activity is first seen in the right
    heart, and the first frame in which activity is seen in the:
    (A) Lungs
    (B) Liver
    (C) Brain
    (D) Inferior vena cava

211. The heart is capable of remodeling in response to environmental burden, and
    a variety of stimuli can induce it to grow or shrink. Which of the following
    conditions can be responsible for developing physiologic hypertrophy?
    (A) Hypertension
    (B) Athletic training
    (C) Bed rest
    (D) Smoking

212. The most frequent cause of false-positive results of Tc-99m sestamibi single isotope dual phase parathyroid scintigraphy is:

    (A) Parathyroid cyst
    (B) Attenuation artifact
    (C) Thyroid nodule
    (D) Thyroiditis

213. F-18 FDG, a radiopharmaceutical for measuring glucose metabolism consists of two components: cyclotron-produced fluorine-18 and a metabolically stable analog of glucose. What is chemical formula of this tracer?

    (A) F-18 chloro-2-deoxy-D-glucose
    (B) F-18 fluoro-2-deoxy-D-glucose
    (C) F-18 fluoro-2-deoxy-L-glucose
    (D) F-18 chloro-2-deoxy-D-glucose

214. Applying Fourier analysis to acquired multiprojection data allows describing images in terms of their spatial frequencies. These are expressed in units:

    (A) Distance/2 (cm/2)
    (B) 1/distance (cm^{-1})
    (C) 1/time (sec^{-1})
    (D) Time/2 (sec/2)

215. The radioactive decay of an atom:

    (A) Is random event
    (B) Results in atom's energy gain
    (C) Correlates with temperature
    (D) Depends on atmospheric pressure

216. Brain natriuretic peptide (BNP), is secreted by the ventricles of the heart in response to excessive stretching of heart muscle cells. The BNP level in the blood is used for diagnosis of:

    (A) Congestive Heart Failure (CHF)
    (B) Hypertension (HTN)
    (C) Supraventricular Tachycardia (SVT)
    (D) Atrial Fibrillation (AFIB)

217. Which of the following characteristic emissions will be most efficiently attenuated by disposable gloves?

    (A) Alpha
    (B) Beta
    (C) Gamma
    (D) X-ray

218. The CRP blood test, or C Reactive Protein test, is one of the essential blood tests in determining risk for developing heart disease. The rise in C Reactive Protein's blood level is an indicator of:
    (A) Hypercoagulation
    (B) Inflammation
    (C) Intoxication
    (D) Hyperlipidemia

219. Displayed below are counts obtained during a HIDA scan with cholecystokinin (CCK) intervention. What is the calculated gallbladder (GB) ejection fraction?

    GB ROI counts prior to CCK administration=81,450 counts in 285 pixel.
    GB ROI counts post-CCK administration=45,359 counts in 214 pixel.
    Background counts prior to CCK administration=4,560 counts in 85 pixel.
    Background counts post-CCK administration=1,582 counts in 85 pixel.
    (A) 37%
    (B) 43%
    (C) 45%
    (D) 53%

220. In medical imaging slices, coinciding with (x, y, z) coordinate system have special names. Axial or transaxial slices lie parallel to the:
    (A) x, z plane
    (B) y, z plane
    (C) x, y plane
    (D) x, y, z plane

Answers

1. C – Coughing helps maintain consciousness
   (AHA Guidelines 2005)

2. B – Heart rate
   (Zaret and Beller 2005)
   Atropine is administered intravenously at the end of 40 µ/kg/min dobutamine infusion in patients who are not able to achieve – e.g., patients using beta blockers – 85% of target heart rate.
   (Mycek and Harvey 2008)

3. A – Photopeak efficiency
   The photopeak efficiency is sensitive to count rate and gamma ray energy.
   (Saha 2006)

4. B – Should be increased
   In adults if the creatinine level is greater than 1.8 mg, the dose of Furosemide should be increased.
   (Sfakianakis et al. 2009)

5. D – The atrioventricular node
   In order to ensure the optimal blood flow, the atrioventricular node slows signal from the sinus node so that the ventricles are not triggered to contract until the atria have fully contracted. The SA node signals the heart to speed up or slow down, and it adjusts its signals according to the body's needs.
   (Podrid 2008)

6. C – Injected patient
   (Oxford Journals 2010)

7. A – Universal System
   The SI system has seven base units – kilogram, meter, seconds, ampere, mole, Kelvin, and candela and two dimensionless units – the radian and the steradian.
   (Wikipedia 2010)

8. A – Quenching
   The addition of a small amount of a polyatomic organic vapor such as butane or ethanol causes collisions of the positive argon ions with the quencher and transfer their charge and some energy to them.
   (Christian 2004)

9. D – 3,400,000 µCi

    (Appendix A, Formula 9A)

10. A – In washout phase

    In the washout phase, the patient is breathing room air from a one-way valve
    through the delivery system and exhaling into the built-in charcoal trap.
    (Saha 2004)

11. D – Alcohols are rapidly germicidal when applied to the skin, but they have no
    appreciable persistent activity
    (CDC Guideline 2002)

12. A – I-123 metaiodobenzylguanidine (MIBG)

    The neurons within the myocardium are more sensitive to the effects of isch-
    emia than the myocytes and the extent of receptor decrease provides prognos-
    tic information that can be used to monitor the response to specific heart failure
    treatment.
    (Cerqueira 2008)

13. B – Geometric efficiency

    The geometric efficiency of the detector decreases with the increased distance
    between the source and the detector and increases with the size of the detector.
    (Saha 2006)

14. A – 0, 1, 2, and 4 h

    Four hours imaging detects more patients with delayed emptying.
    (Odunsi and Camilleri 2009)

15. C – Akinetic left ventricle

    Akinesis – seen there on the anteroapical surfaces – refers to absent contractile
    function of the left ventricle, e.g., after a heart attack. The heart muscle in the
    distribution of the involved vessels is often akinetic due to the lack or dimin-
    ished blood supply.
    (Zaret and Beller 2005)

16. B – Diagnostic imaging

    (Medscape Radiology 2010)

17. C – A particle having a mass equal to the electron but opposite charge
    (Early and Sodee 1995)

18. B – Blunders

Systematic errors relate to the method of observation, e.g., malfunctioning well counter. Random errors relate to the event being observed, e.g., radioactive decay.
(Lombardi 1999)

19. D – 138

(Appendix A, Formula 12)

20. D – Labeled erythrocytes scintigraphy

A technetium-labeled red blood cell scintigraphy is used in the evaluation of gastrointestinal bleeding. A PET using F-18 FDG has become an important diagnostic tool in patients with FUO.
(Bleeker-Rovers et al. 2009)

21. D – When chyme enters the intestine

Chyme is the thick semifluid mass of partially digested food that passes from the stomach to the duodenum. The rate of gastric emptying is strongly influenced by both volume and composition of gastric contents (liquid vs. solid).
(Frohlich 2001)

22. A – High sensitivity and low specificity

A bone scan is used as a routine screening tool for staging in numbers of cancers and in many benign musculoskeletal conditions because of its low cost, sensitivity, availability, and the ability to scan entire skeleton.
(Gnanasegaran et al. 2009)

23. A – The relative error

Relative error formula is applied:
Relative error $= (x - x_0)/x$
Where, $x =$ true value of a quantity,
$x_0 =$ observed value of the quantity,
$x - x_0 =$ absolute error.
(Lombardi 1999)

24. B – Fracture with history of trauma

Irregular distribution in the axial skeleton and ribs is typical for bone metastases.
(Gnanasegaran et al. 2009)

25. B – Inferior portion of the heart

The left anterior descending supplies blood to the anterior heart and the septum. The circumflex supplies the posterior portion of the left ventricle. The right coronary artery supplies the bottom portion of the ventricles.
(Christian et al. 2004)

26. C – F-18 fluoride exposure is 70% higher than Tc99m exposure
     (SNM guideline 2010)

27. A – An electron
     (Early and Sodee 1995)

28. A – RAM
     RAM – random access memory – its volatile information contents is lost when,
     e.g., the electric power to the computer is switched off.
     (Christian et al. 2004)

29. A – 36.7 ml
     (Appendix A, Formula 36B)

30. B – Flare phenomenon
     A super scan is characterized by excellent bone detail and is observed in the
     diffuse metastatic process when virtually all of the radiotracer is concentrated
     in the skeleton, with little or no activity in the soft tissues or urinary tract.
     (Gnanasegaran et al. 2009)

31. B – Pulmonary veins
     (Early and Sodee 1995)

32. A – Radiation pneumonitis
     Pulmonary uptake can also be seen in patients with malignant pleural effusion
     and hyperparathyroidism.
     (Gnanasegaran et al. 2009)

33. C – Enhances low counts
     A logarithmic relationship assigns more levels to low count pixels and com-
     presses the number of shades assigned to high pixel values.
     (Christian et al. 2004)

34. D – Magnetic resonance imaging-magnetic activity
     Confirmatory examinations, including imaging tests, may be called on in special
     situations to supplement the physical examination when specific components
     cannot be reliably performed or evaluated.
     (Zuckier and Kolano 2008)

35. D – 5.9 mCi of Tc-99m Mebrofenin
     (Christian et al. 2004)

36. B – The number performed of cardiac imaging procedures increased
    (Mettler et al. 2008)

37. A – Isomers
    (Early and Sodee 1995)

38. D – Direct memory access (DMA)
    Direct memory access takes the CPU out of the loop for data acquisition allow-
    ing very high counts rate to be stored.
    (Christian et al. 2004)

39. A – 78,000 rems
    (Appendix A, Formula 9D)

40. B – Is characterized by rapid blood clearance
    A radiolabeled sulfur colloid is rapidly cleared from the vascular space by
    extraction to liver, spleen, and bone marrow and successful visualization of the
    bleeding site depends on active bleeding occurring within a time-window of
    several minutes after radiotracer administration.
    (Howarth 2006)

41. B – Negative feedback
    When levels of T_3 and T_4 are high, TSH production is decreased and when the
    levels of T_3 and T_4 are low, the production of TSH is increased. This effect cre-
    ates a regulatory negative feedback loop.
    (Frohlich 2001)

42. C – Patients selection
    The results of Tc-99m-labeled red blood cell scintigraphy are highly dependent
    on both the appropriate selection of the patient and correct timing of the test.
    Careful selection of patients to include those who have a high likelihood of
    active bleeding greatly increases the clinical utility of these tests.
    (Howarth 2006)

43. C – WC counts activity within the patient, UP counts patient samples
    (Early and Sodee 1995)

44. D – Is misinterpreted as breast attenuation artifact
    (Gnanasegaran et al. 2009)

45. C – A anterior and B posterior view
    The cardiac silhouette is more prominent on the anterior projection
    (Christian et al. 2004)

46. A – Effective dose
     (CDC glossary 2010)

47. D – Procedure type
     The patient's own medical conditions such as failure of hepatobiliary and geni-
     tourinary systems; dose infiltration and even simple conditions, such as exces-
     sive talking can alter radiopharmaceutical biodistribution.
     (Vallabhajosula et al. 2010)

48. A – Horizontal and vertical line straightness
     (Christian 2004)

49. A – 55 h
     (Appendix A, Formula 18)

50. A – Fistulous connection is present
     (Gnanasegaran et al. 2009)

51. A – Catecholamines
     Adrenal medulla is the body's main source of the circulating catecholamines
     adrenaline (epinephrine) and noradrenaline (norepinephrine).
     (Early and Sodee 1995)

52. B – Photopenic area
     (Zaret and Beller 2005)

53. D – Reproducibility, uniformity, and blank scan
     Reproducibility is one of the main principles of the counting statistics, and
     refers to the ability of a test or experiment to be accurately replicated, by some-
     one else working independently. Blank scan is performed daily in PET.
     (Early and Sodee 1995)

54. B – Surgical incision wounds
     Surgical wounds are healing by first intention (primary union), restoration of
     tissue continuity occurs directly, without granulation.
     (Love and Palestro 2010)

55. C – 6.1 mCi of Tc-99m Sulfur colloid
     A liver–spleen scan with sulfur colloid allows interpreting physician to assess
     the size, shape, and position of the liver and spleen and to detect, measure, and
     monitor masses of the liver and/or spleen.
     (Christian 2004)

56. C – Dehydrated

Dehydration is defined as an excessive loss of body fluid caused by losing too much fluid and/or not drinking. Vomiting and diarrhea are common causes. The elderly and those with illnesses are at higher risk of dehydration. (Christian 2004)

57. D – Radiochemical purity

The presence of free Tc-99m pertechnetate in Tc-99m radiopharmaceuticals is a common example of radiochemical impurity. (Saha 2006)

58. B – Hounsfield Unit

Each voxel is assigned a value on a scale in which air has a value of −1,000; water, 0; kidney 30, and compact bone, +1,000. (Wahl 2009)

59. C – 8%

(Appendix A, Formula 10A)

60. C – Activated neutrophils adhere to the pulmonary capillaries for a longer period than do nonactivated neutrophils

(Love and Palestro 2010)

61. B – QT interval

(Podrid 2008)

62. A – Stimulates uptake of leukocytes but suppresses uptake of sulfur colloid

(Love and Palestro 2010)

63. C – 5%

(ASNC Information Statement 2010)

64. A – The hemorrhage cessation

The results of scintigraphy are highly dependent on both the appropriate selection of the patient and correct timing of the test. (Howarth 2006)

65. A – Tc-99-labeled RBCs and Tc-99m sulfur colloid

(Christian et al. 2004)

66. C – Deliver higher effective dose to the patient

(Stein et al. 2007)

67. A – Thyroid imaging

(Saha 2006)

68. B – Scatter correction

In this method, the coincidence events are accumulated in two separate energy windows. The dual-window technique makes the assumption that scattered photons collected in the lower than photopeak energy window are linearly proportional to the scattered photons in the photopeak window.
(Christian et al. 2004)

69. A – 5.0 mCi

(Appendix A, Formula 25)

70. C – Delay imaging

(Ziessman 2009)

71. C – Lipids

Steroids are lipids that contain four carbon ring joined to form the steroid nucleus. Examples of steroids include cholesterol, the sex hormones estradiol and testosterone, and the anti-inflammatory drug dexamethasone.
(Wikipedia 2010)

72. B – 1.0–1.5 min

(ASNC Imaging Guidelines 2006)

73. C – Random events correction

Since the delayed window includes only the random events and the standard window contains true and random events, correction is being made by subtracting the delay window from the standard window.
(Saha 2005)

74. D – Blood pool

(Wahl 2009)

75. D – Palmar view

(Frohlich 2001)

76. C – Cardiac CT

(Radiologyinfo.com 2010)

77. B – Are taken up by the cells of RES in liver and spleen

Aluminum phosphate coprecipitates also with a Tc-99m Sc and the particles are trapped in the lung capillaries.

(Vallabhajosula et al. 2010)

78. C – Xe-133

Xenon 133 gas is for diagnostic inhalation use only and cannot be detected on the surfaces.

(Early and Sodee 1995)

79. A – 18.2 mCi

No need to obtain concentration, just decay 22.7 mCi to 35 min to get correct answer.

(Appendix A, Formula 25)

80. A – Overestimated

The CT data with energies of 70–140 keV used for the purpose of PET attenuation correction in combined PET/CT are attenuated considerably more by structures that contain elements with high atomic numbers, such as iodine and barium.

(Lin and Alavi 2009)

81. B – Melena-black tarry stool

Hematopoiesis – the normal formation and development of blood cells in the bone marrow; hemosiderosis – an increased deposition of iron in a selection of tissues.

(Mosby 1998)

82. D – Urinary Tract Infection (UTI)

Disseminated intravascular coagulation (DIC) is a pathological activation of blood clotting mechanisms in response to a variety of diseases and leads to the formation of small blood clots inside the blood vessels throughout the body.

(Stein et al. 2007)

83. A – Produces centers of luminescence

Interactions of X-rays or gamma rays will not induce light from crystal of pure NaI.

(Christian et al. 2004)

84. D – Dose extravasation

(Zaret and Beller 2005)

85. B – Rib fractures

A delay of several days should be allowed after an acute trauma to increase the sensitivity of radionuclear imaging for rib fracture visualization. (Early and Sodee 1999)

86. A – Negative air pressure (Early and Sodee 1995)

87. A – Arise from the breakdown of the material

Additives and/or buffers are not impurities. (Saha 2006)

88. B – Acquisition time

Narrow energy window, high-energy photons and narrow FWHM will produce less scatter. (Early and Sodee 1999)

89. B – 3.6 mCi (Appendix A, Formula 26)

90. B – Inspecting the rotating planar images (Zaret and Beller 2005)

91. B – The hepatic flexure to the splenic flexure (Frohlich 1993)

92. C – Septal, inferoapical, and lateral walls

The anterior view provides information regarding contraction of the apical and anterior segments. Multiple views are necessary since in a planar technique cardiac and noncardiac structures can obscure ROI. (Zaret and Beller 2005)

93. C – Sum peaks

Summing of pulses from multiple photon interactions is called pulse pileup. (Consultants in Nuclear Medicine 2010)

94. A – Flickering (Zaret and Beller 2005)

95. D – Horizontal long axis (Zaret and Beller 2005)

96. A – Alpha particles

Leaf tobacco contains diminutive amounts of lead Pb-210 and alpha particle-emitting polonium-210 both of which are radioactive carcinogens and both of which can be found in smoke from burning tobacco.
(Wikipedia 2010)

97. C – Rubidium-82

(Christian et al. 2004)

98. B – Sinogram

The sinogram – image representation of raw data obtained when projection–reconstruction imaging is used.
(Christian et al. 2004)

99. C – 11.2 mCi

(Appendix A, Formula 25)

100. B – Roll-off

At coronary blood flow levels exceeding 2.5 ml/min/g the radiotracers show a significant roll-off. The roll-off is the smallest for Tl-201 and is larger for ^{99m}Tc-99m sestamibi and ^{99m}Tc-99m tetrofosmin.
(Zaret and Beller 2005)

101. B – Increased high-density lipoprotein (HDL) cholesterol

Elevated plasma homocysteine can injure endothelium which can lead to thromboembolic events and arteriosclerosis.
(Andreoli et al. 2001)

102. A – Underestimation of the ES volume

(Zaret and Beller 2005)

103. B – Dead-time counting losses

Dead-time counting losses result in counting-rate-related image degradation.
(Zanzonico 2008)

104. B – 68

Each segment the 17-segment model is scored on a 5-point scale: 0=normal, 1=slight reduction of tracer uptake (ambivalent), 2=moderate reduction of uptake (typically implies a significant abnormality), 3=harsh reduction of uptake, and 4=absence of uptake.
(Zaret and Beller 2005)

105. C – Carcinoid tumor

OctreoScan binds to somatostatin receptors in tissues throughout the body, but concentrates in tumors that contain a higher density of somatostatin receptors. Primary carcinoid tumor of the liver are extremely rare but about 75% of all carcinoid tumors metastasize to the liver.
(Medscape Today 2010)

106. C – Direct effect of radiation
(EPA 2010)

107. B – Binding energy
(Early and Sodee 1995)

108. B – At least two quadrants

With the new cameras on the market, at least a segment of the lead bars 2.5-mm wide should be visible as well.
(Zanzonico 2008)

109. D – 113 mCi

Obtain precalibration of given activity for each different time given in the problem and add all three precalibrated activity answers to obtain accumulative activity needed. Precalibration activity is always more than activity given; therefore, depending on the half-life answer could be estimated.
(Appendix A, Formula 25)

110. A – Left Anterior Descending (LAD)

The data show that the average defect size is larger in isolated LAD than in isolated LCX or RCA.
(Iskandrian and Verani 2003)

111. C – Liver

Gall bladder, spleen, stomach, small bowel, transverse, ascending, and descending colon also lie in the intraperitoneal space.
(Wikipedia 2010)

112. C – Chest pain

Patients undergoing stress testing with adenosine most frequently experienced flushing followed closely by dyspnea and chest pain.
(Zaret and Beller 2005)

113. B – Gas-filled radiation detectors
(Early and Sodee 1995)

114. B – Renal scintigraphy

MAG3 has high overall extraction efficiency (EE) of approximately 60%. MAG3 is mainly a tubular agent allowing the cortex imaging even when the GFR is minimal or absent.

(Sfakianakis et al. 2009)

115. D – Autonomously hyperfunctioning thyroid nodule

The presence of autonomously hyperfunctioning thyroid nodule has been associated in some instances with thyrotoxicosis; however, many patients with nodules sufficiently hyperactive have been found to be clinically euthyroid.

(Early and Sodee 1995)

116. A – 50 mrem/month

(Consultants in Nuclear Medicine 2010)

117. D – Excitation

(Early and Sodee 1995)

118. A – Spatial frequencies above a cutoff frequency

Low-pass filters eliminate spatial frequencies above a cutoff frequency and thus reduce noise.

(Groch and Erwin 2000)

119. C – 2.7 ml

Answer of Formula 29 should be subtracted from volume needed (4 ml) to get desired volume.

(Appendix A, Formula 29)

120. B – Cold spot

Vena cava obstruction due to lung cancer can appear as a hot spot on the liver–spleen scan. Patchy areas can be present in lacerations and advanced cirrhosis.

(Christian 2004)

121. C – The brain

At the base of the brain, the carotid and vertebrobasilar arteries form a circle of communicating arteries known as the circle of Willis.

(Frohlich 1993)

122. A – Neuroblastoma

The adrenal medulla and the neural crest are the most common affected organs of the primary neuroblastoma.

(Grünwald and Ezziddin 2010)

123. A – The absence of any material in the FOV
(Zanzonico 2008)

124. A – B cells

Approximately 85% of lymphomas that occur in the USA and Western Europe are derived from B cells and are for this reason known as B-cell lymphomas. (Goldsmith 2010)

125. A – Irreversible defect

The irreversible or the fixed defect is a defect that is unchanged and present on both exercise and rest images. This pattern commonly is sign of the presence of myocardial infarction and scar tissue. In our case the polar plot display indicates presence of large, irreversible defect involving the cardiac apex. (Christian et al. 2004)

126. C – Tl-201 stress-reinjection
(ASNC Information 2010)

127. A – Photon mass is equal to electron mass
(Early and Sodee 1995)

128. B – LeVeen shunt

Peritoneal–venous shunt used in the control of ascites caused by cirrhosis of the liver, right-sided heart failure, or abdominal cancer. (Early and Sodee 1995)

129. D – 7.5 mCi
(Appendix A, Formula 31A)

130. C – Salvage therapy
(NCI 2010)

131. A – The spleen
(Early and Sodee 1995)

132. A – A chimeric monoclonal antibody to a tumor antigen
Chimeric monoclonal antibody is made from human and mouse proteins. (Goldsmith 2010)

133. B – Collimator integrity
(Eradimaging 2010)

134. B – To confirm normal biodistribution of the labeled antibody

In the USA, the FDA requires intravenous administration of In-111 ibritu-momab at the time of the initial rituximab infusion and whole-body scanning 24–72 h later. It is required that the whole-body image, anterior and posterior views, is examined to confirm normal biodistribution.
(Goldsmith 2010)

135. B – Cystic duct

The cystic duct is the short duct – 2 to 3 cm in length – that joins the gall blad-der to the common bile duct.
(Early and Sodee 1995)

136. B – Require further validation
(ASNC Information 2010)

137. D – Drug interaction
(Gnanasegaran et al. 2009)

138. C – Lower resolution, higher sensitivity
(Early and Sodee 1995)

139. C – 0.07 µCi Mo-99/mCi Tc-99m
(Appendix A, Formula 30B)

140. A – A human IgG sequence
(Goldsmith 2010)

141. D – 12

The remaining vertebrae: cervical 7, lumbar 5, five that are fused to form the sacrum and the four coccygeal bones that form the tailbone.
(Frohlich 1993)

142. C – Recent (within 1–2 weeks) liver function tests
(Goldsmith 2010)

143. A – Septal penetration
(Early and Sodee 1995)

144. D – Too large

The particle size of a radiopharmaceutical greatly affects its biokinetics, e.g., a particle size of less than 0.1 µm is necessary for migration from the injection site and uptake into the lymph nodes.
(Vallabhajosula et al. 2010)

145. A – Dilated nonobstructed pattern

Kidneys show gradually increasing activity followed by washout after Lasix administration.

(Christian et al. 2004)

146. B – Recordable event

(Nuclear Medicine Tutorials 2010)

147. C – Electron capture

(Early and Sodee 1995)

148. D – Increased the apparent size of the object

(Early and Sodee 1995)

149. D – 2.7 h

(Appendix A, Formula 30C)

150. D – The sentinel node

(Christian et al. 2004)

151. A – Methimazole and Propylthiouracil

Besides antithyroid drugs and radioiodine treatment, surgery with subtotal thyroidectomy is the treatment of choice for patients with obstructive symptoms.

(Andreoli et al. 1997)

152. D – Radiolabeled macroaggregated human albumin

In patients with pulmonary hypertension (PH) the numbers of injected particles should be reduced in proportion to the severity of the PH; in infants and children that number is adjusted according to weight. The pregnant patient receives the administered dose reduced to half of the usual dose.

(Bailey et al. 2010)

153. C – Fourier transform

(Christian et al. 2004)

154. A – Is a normal variation

The thyroid gland is a butterfly-shape organ and is composed of two wing-like lobes: right and left lobe united via the narrow isthmus.

(Smith and Oates 2004)

155. B – Hepatocytes

After intravenous injection, IDA derivates are rapidly bound to plasma albumin, circulate to the liver, where they dissociate from their binding albumins and are taken up by the hepatocytes in a manner similar to bilirubin, reaching peak activity in the liver in 12 min. The liver uptake is influenced by plasma albumin concentration, hepatic blood flow, and hepatocyte functions. Note the nonvisualization of gallbladder at 2-h.

(Christian et al. 2004)

156. A – Stochastic effects

(U.S. Environmental Protection Agency 2010)

157. B – Pb collimator

The photoelectric (PE) is most present if the Z number of the absorbing medium is high.

(Christian et al. 2004)

158. C – TP requires a lead collimator

A cylindrical, 20–29 cm long, lead collimator covers the probe and the photo-multiplier (PM) tube.

(Saha 2006)

159. A – Between 24,193 and 24,819 cpm

(Appendix A, Formula 13)

160. B – Increases with the nodule size

Nodule size >2.5 cm can cause toxicity, and the suppression of the remainder of the gland implies autonomy of the nodule.

(Smith and Oates 2004)

161. C – 45%

The normal range is between 37 and 47% in women and between 40 and 54% in men.

(Perry and Potter 2006)

162. C – 150–200 mCi

For postoperative ablation of thyroid remnants 75–150 mCi and for treatment of distant metastases >200 mCi are typically administered.

(SNM Guideline 2002)

163. B – Well counter

Placing the source in the central hole of the detector, e.g., well counter or dose calibrator increases the detector geometric efficiency close to 99%.
(Saha 2006)

164. A – Quantitative measurements of bone remodeling

Quantitative measurements of bone remodeling have an important role in research studies examining the pathophysiology of metabolic bone diseases and the response of patients to treatment.
(Moore et al. 2008)

165. A – Right renal pelvis

The renal pelvis is located at the center of the kidney and is described as enlarged upper end of the ureter.
(Christian et al. 2004)

166. C – FedEx

Nuclear Regulatory Commission (NRC) and The States can also develop these rules.
(NRC 2010)

167. D – Iron

They have the same oxidation state and comparable ionic radius.
(Christian et al. 2004)

168. D – Dead time settings
(Saha 2006)

169. D – 12 ft
(Appendix A, Formula 16)

170. C – Pelvis and lumbar spine

Paget's disease of bone is a chronic disorder of the skeleton in which areas of bone undergo abnormal turnover, leading to areas of enlarged and softened bone.
(Chaffins 2007)

171. C – Salvage therapy
(NCI 2010)

172. C – Continuous

The smaller the arc used for each projection, the less blurring from the camera motion.

(Christian et al. 2004)

173. A – The number of ionizations is converted to curie (Ci) or becquerel (Bq)

A dose calibrator is an ionization chamber. Rad or gray are units of the absorbed dose; biological risk is estimated using the conventional unit rem or sievert.

(Christian et al. 2004)

174. A – The sympathetic activity

A I-123 metaiodobenzylguanidine (MIBG) is a radiopharmaceutical with properties that allow evaluating, e.g., the differences in myocardial sympathetic innervations.

(Christian et al. 2004)

175. A – Cold nodule

Thyroid nodules increase with age and are present in almost 10% of the adult population. The majority (~85%) of cold nodules are benign-cold nodules are more commonly evaluated to make sure they do not represent malignancy.

(Christian et al. 2004)

176. C – Jelly wastes

Generators eluants, radiopharmaceuticals in vials, leftovers of kits etc. are liquid wastes.

(Lombardi 1999)

177. D – I-131

Iodine-131, also called radioiodine, is a radioisotope of iodine and it is a major uranium fission product.

(Christian et al. 2004)

178. B – Sentinel node

Intraoperative probes are highly collimated counting devices, e.g., solid-state scintillation or ionization detectors.

(Zanzonico 2008)

179. A – 6.3 mR/h

Since each HVL reduces exposure to half, simply divide 25 by 2 twice to achieve the answer.

(Appendix A, Formula 17)

180. D – Stress electrocardiography

An exercise EKG is a test that checks for electrocardiogram abnormalities during exercise. This test is sometimes called a "stress test" or a "treadmill test." (Wahl 2009)

181. A – Diastole

During diastole the pressure within the myocardium is lower than that in aorta, allowing blood to circulate in the heart itself via the coronary arteries. (Vitola and Delbeke 2004)

182. C – Dobutamine

Esmolol decreases the force and rate of heart contractions induced by dobutamine infusion by blocking beta-adrenergic receptors in the heart. (Vitola and Delbeke 2004)

183. C – The signature of lead technologist

The results of the test and comments indicating if the test was or was not acceptable should be also included in the test documents. (Zanzonico 2008)

184. D – Sm-153

It emits a gamma ray photon of 103 keV that is appropriate for nuclear medicine imaging. (Saha 2004)

185. C – Right posterior oblique and left posterior oblique

Note the lack of heart shadow which is not present on posterior views of normal lung perfusion scans. Planar images should be obtained in multiple projections, including anterior, posterior, and both posterior oblique. (Christian et al. 2004)

186. A – Emits light after heating

Thermoluminescence crystals when exposed to gamma- or X-rays and then heated, emit flashes of light with intensity proportional to the absorbed dose. (Lombardi 1999)

187. B – Are positively or negatively charged electrons

(Early and Sodee 1995)

188. C – Monthly high-count floods

Manufacturer's references vary, although a usual acquisition is in the range of 100 million counts for a large field-of-view camera acquired monthly. (Zanzonico 2008)

189. A – 97%

Subtract background counts from all given counts

(Appendix A, Formula 32A)

190. C – Data base normal study of an age and gender matched population

(Zaret and Beller 2005)

191. B – Goitrogens

Chemicals, drugs and food that have been shown to have goitrogenic effects include, e.g., thiocyanate, amiodarone, lithium, carbamazepine, peanuts, and gluten.

(Wikipedia 2010)

192. C – <0.44

The demonstration of increased lung uptake on MPI SPECT postexercise images serves as a marker of severe and extensive CAD and reduced left ventricular function.

(Zaret and Beller 2005)

193. A – Co-56 and Co-58

22 radioisotopes have been characterized with the most stable Co-60 with a half-life of 5.2714 years, Co-57 (271.79 days), Co-56 (77.27 days), and Co-58 (70.86 days). All of the left behind have half-lives that are less than 18 h and the bulk of these have half-lives that are less than 1 s.

194. C – Cutoff values for an abnormal TID ratio vary

The values of the TID index are dependent on acquisition protocol, patient gender, type of stressor, processing technique, software used, etc.

(Zaret and Beller 2005)

195. C – External transmission source

The transmission image helps define the position of the sentinel node. The sentinel lymph node is potentially the first node to receive the lymph-borne metastatic cells. Lymphoscintigraphy allows the surgeon to easily identify and biopsy the sentinel lymph node.

(Shackett 2008)

196. B – Ga-67 citrate

Whole body dose from Ga-67citrate –0.260 rad/mCi; Tl-201 chloride-0.210 rad/mCi; F-18 FDG –0.040 rad/mCi; Tc-99m-0.017 rad/mCi

(Lombardi 1999)

197. B – Isobars
      (Saha 2004)

198. B – Collimator
      (Early and Sodee 1995)

199. A – 26%
      (Appendix A, Formula 35B)

200. B – 16-frame gating localizes end systole frame more precisely
      (Zaret and Beller 2005)

201. C – Early bystander CPR
      Early recognition of the emergency and activation of the emergency medical
      services is the first link in the Chain of Survival followed by early CPR. CPR
      plus defibrillation within 3–5 min of collapse can produce survival rates as
      high as 49–75%. Early advanced life support followed by postresuscitation
      care delivered by healthcare providers is the last link in the chain.
      (AHA 2010)

202. D – Vascularity of involved of tissue
      Blood pool images show the level of soft tissue involvement, and delayed
      images indicate osteoblastic response to the underlying disease.
      (Christian 2004)

203. A – Loss of detail
      (Groch 2000)

204. B – Masking technique
      In some patients, SPECT imaging is helpful to better characterize the pres-
      ence, location, and extent of disease.
      (Christian 2004)

205. C – Hematoma of the thigh
      CT scan-Fig. 3.21a revealed presence of large hematoma (arrow) within the
      posterior muscles of the right thigh extending from the level of ischium
      through to the level just above the knee and measuring approx. 27 cm.
          The most well-known clinical indications of red blood cells scintigraphy
      are to localize lower gastrointestinal bleeding, to diagnose hepatic heman-
      giomas and to calculate LVEF (Muga scan). There are descriptions in the
      literature of RBC scan application for evaluation of active bleeding in soft
      tissues.

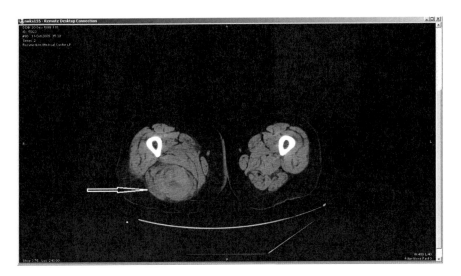

Fig. 3.22 CT scan

206. C – Bladder

The bladder receives 0.440 rad/mCi but the radiation dose varies with patient hydration and voiding frequency. Critical organ is the organ most vulnerable to a given radiopharmaceutical due to increased susceptibility for malignancy and limits the dose of the radiopharmaceutical.

(Early and Sodee 1995)

207. A – Tc-99m MAG3

A Tc-99m MAG is presently the agent of choice because of lower radiation dose to the patient and better photon energy of Tc-99m when compared to I-131 or a I-123 Hippuran. A Tc-99m DMSA is a cortical imaging agent (40–50% fixed to cortex).

(Sfakianakis 2009)

208. A – Colorimetric test

The presence of aluminum can be detected by the colorimetric method using aurin tricarboxylic acid or methyl orange, and can be quantified by comparison with a standard solution of aluminum.

(Saha 2004)

209. D – 7%

(Appendix A, Formula 10A)

210. A – Lungs

When drawing the region of interest (ROI) over the right ventricle careful attention should be paid to the separation between the right atrium (RA) and RV.
(Zaret and Beller 2005)

211. B – Athletic training

Physiologic hypertrophy is a compensatory change in the proportion and function of the heart.
(Cohn 2006)

212. C – Thyroid nodule

Other possible causes of F (+) results include a Tc-99m Sestamibi accumulation in thyroid carcinoma and lymphadenopathy.
(Palestro et al. 2005)

213. B – F-18 fluoro-2-deoxy-D-glucose
(Lin and Alavi 2009)

214. B – 1/distance (cm^{-1})

In Fourier space image subtle detail is associated with higher frequencies, and coarser structures with lower frequencies.
(Christian 2004)

215. A – Is random event

Radioactive decay is the spontaneous breakdown of an atomic nucleus resulting in the release of energy and matter from the nucleus.
(Early and Sodee 1995)

216. A – CHF

Congestive heart failure is caused by myocardial infarction, CAD, or cardiomyopathy and is characterized by the failure of the ventricle to eject blood resourcefully resulting in volume overload and chamber dilatation.
(Family Health Guide 2010)

217. A – Alpha

Because of their mass and low velocity, alpha particles are very likely to interact with other atoms and lose their energy, so their forward motion is effectively stopped within a few centimeters of air.
(Early and Sodee 1995)

218. B – *Inflammation*

The rise of CRP is due to an increase in the plasma concentration of interleukin which is produced predominantly by macrophages as well as adipocytes. (Mosby 1998)

219. A – 37%

Net ROI counts should be obtained using formula 33 – Net ROI counts. If net ROI counts are given then just use formula 34 only.

(Appendix A, Formula 33 and 34)

220. C – *x, y* plane

The expected products of SPECT are images that represent cross-sectional slices of the body perpendicular to the imaging table or parallel to *x, y* plane. (Christian 2004)

References and Suggested Readings

American Heart Association Guidelines for Cardiopulmonary Resuscitation and Emergency Cardiovascular Care. Circulation. http://circ.ahajournals.org/cgi/content/full/112/24_suppl/ IV-47. Accessed 11 Apr 2007.

Andreoli TE, Bennett JC, et al. Cecil essentials of medicine. 5th ed. Philadelphia, PA: WB Saunders; 2001.

ASNC Information Statement. Recommendations for reducing radiation exposure in myocardial perfusion imaging. http://www.asnc.org/imageuploads/RadiationReduction060110.pdf. Accessed 23 Aug 2010.

Bailey AE, Bailey LD, Roach JP. V/Q imaging in 2010: a quick start guide. Semin Nucl Med. 2010;40:408–14.

Bleeker-Rovers CP, Van der Meer JWM, Oyen WJG. Fever of unknown origin. Semin Nucl Med. 2009;39:81–7.

Braunwald L et al. Harrison's principles of internal medicine. 15th ed. New York, NY: McGraw-Hill; 2001.

CDC. Emergency Preparedness and Response. Glossary. http://www.bt.cdc.gov/radiation/glossary. asp. Accessed 28 Aug 2010.

CDC. Guideline for Hand Hygiene in Health-Care Settings. http://www.cdc.gov/mmwr/PDF/rr/ rr5116.pdf. Accessed 21 June 2010.

Cerqueira M. Beyond SPECT Perfusion: New Radiotracers for Imaging Cardiac Sympathetic Innervation. Metabolism and PET Perfusion. http://cme.medscape.com/viewarticle/582783. Accessed 10 Dec 2008.

Christian PE, Bernier DR, Langan JK. Nuclear medicine and PET: technology and techniques. 5th ed. St. Louis, MO: Mosby; 2004.

Cohn JN. Cardiac remodeling: basic aspects. Official reprint from UpToDate. www.uptodate.com. Accessed 19 Apr 2006.

Consultants in Nuclear Medicine. Karesh P. http://www.nucmedconsultants.com. Accessed 7 June 2010.

Early PJ, Sodee BD. Principles and practice of nuclear medicine. 2nd ed. St. Louis, MO: Mosby; 1995.

Eradimaging. Nuclear Medicine Instrumentation and Quality Control: A Review. http://eradimaging. com/site/article.cfm?ID=88&mode=ce. Accessed 28 Oct 2010.

Family Health Guide. Harvard Medical School. http://www.health.harvard.edu/fhg/updates/BNP-An-important-new-cardiac-test.shtml Accessed 22 Sept 2010

Frohlich ED. Rypin's basic sciences review. 18th ed. Philadelphia, PA: J. B. Lippincott Company; 2001.

Gnanasegaran G, Gary CG, Adamson K, Fogelman I. Patterns, variants, artifacts, and pitfalls in conventional radionuclide bone imaging and SPECT/CT. Semin Nucl Med. 2009;39:380–95.

Goldsmith SJ. Radioimmunotherapy of lymphoma: bexxar and zevalin. Semin Nucl Med. 2010;40:122–35.

Groch MW, Erwin WD. SPECT in the year 2000: basic principles. J Med Technol. 2000;4:233–44.

Grünwald F, Ezziddin S. 131I-Metaiodobenzylguanidine therapy of neuroblastoma and other neuroendocrine tumors. Semin Nucl Med. 2010;40:153–63.

Howarth DM. The role of nuclear medicine in the detection of acute gastrointestinal bleeding. Semin Nucl Med. 2006;36:133–46.

ICRP. Pregnancy and Medical Radiation. www.icrp.org/downloadDoc.asp?document=docs/ICRP_84. Accessed 14 Aug 2010.

Iskandrian AE, Verani MS. Nuclear cardiac imaging: principles and applications. 3rd ed. New York, NY: Oxford University Press; 2003.

Kassis AI. Therapeutic radionuclides: biophysical and radiobiologic principles. Semin Nucl Med. 2008;38:358–66.

Lin CE, Alavi A. PET and PET/CT: a clinical guide. 2nd ed. New York, NY: Thieme; 2009.

Lombardi MH. Radiation safety in nuclear medicine. Boca Raton, FL: CRC; 1999.

Love C, Palestro CJ. Altered biodistribution and incidental findings on gallium and labeled leukocyte/bone marrow scans. Semin Nucl Med. 2010;40(4):271–82.

Medscape Radiology. Radiation Imaging: Slideshow. http://www.medscape.com/features/slideshow/radiation-imaging?src=ptalk&uac=94641PJ. Accessed 20 June 2010.

Medscape Today. Scintigraphic Evaluation of Neuroendocrine Tumors: Indium-111 OctreoScan. http://www.medscape.com/viewarticle/406655_3. Accessed 13 Nov 2010.

Mettler FA, Guiberteau MJ. Essentials of nuclear medicine imaging. 5th ed. Philadelphia, PA: Saunders Elsevier; 2006.

Mettler FA, Bhargavan M, et al. Nuclear medicine exposure in the United States, 2005–2007: preliminary results. Semin Nucl Med. 2008;38(5):384–91.

Moore AEB, Blake GM, Fogelman I. Quantitative measurements of bone remodeling using 99mTc-methylene diphosphonate bone scans and blood sampling. J Nucl Med. 2008;49:375–82.

Mosby Inc. Mosby's medical, nursing & allied health dictionary. 5th ed. St. Louis, MO: Mosby; 1998.

Mycek MJ, Harvey RA. Lippincott's illustrated reviews: pharmacology. 3rd ed. Philadelphia, PA: Lippincott; 2008.

NCI. Dictionary of Cancer Terms. http://www.cancer.gov/dictionary/. Accessed 15 Oct 2010.

Nuclear Medicine Tutorials. http://www.nucmedtutorials.com/dwnrc/nrc2-1.html. Accessed 7 June 2010.

Odunsi ST, Camilleri M. Selected interventions in nuclear medicine: gastrointestinal motor functions. Semin Nucl Med. 2009;39:186–94.

Oxford Journals. Radiation Protection Dosimetry. Radiation exposure of patients and personnel from a PET/CT procedure with F-18 FDG. http://rpd.oxfordjournals.org/content/early/2010/02/18/rpd.ncq026.abstract. Accessed 28 Aug 2010.

Palestro JC, Tomas BM, Tronco GG. Radionuclide imaging of the parathyroid glands. Semin Nucl Med. 2005;35:266–76.

Perry AG, Potter PA. Clinical nursing skills and techniques. 7th ed. St. Louis, MO: Mosby Elsevier; 2006.

Podrid PJ. ECG tutorial. Official reprint from UpToDate. www.uptodate.com. Accessed 05 May 2008.

Radiologyinfo.com. Cardiac CT for Calcium Scoring. http://www.radiologyinfo.org/. Accessed 24 Sept 2010.

Saha GB. Fundamentals of nuclear pharmacy. 5th ed. New York, NY: Springer; 2004.

Saha GB. Basics of PET imaging. New York, NY: Springer; 2005.

Saha GB. Physics and radiobiology of nuclear medicine. 3rd ed. New York, NY: Springer; 2006.

Sfakianakis G, Sfakianaki E, Georgiu M, et al. A renal protocol for all ages and all indications: mercapto-acetyl-triglycine (MAG3) with simultaneous injection of Furosemide (MAG3-F0): a 17-year experience. Semin Nucl Med. 2009;39(3):156–73.

Shackett P. Nuclear medicine technology: procedure and quick reference. 2nd ed. Philadelphia, PA: Lippincott Williams & Wilkins; 2008.

Smith J, Oates E. Radionuclide imaging of the thyroid gland: patterns, pearls, and pitfalls. Clin Nucl Med. 2004;29:181–93.

SNM. Procedure guideline for therapy of thyroid disease with iodine-131. J Nucl Med. 2002;43(6):856–61.

SNM Guideline for Sodium F-18 Fluoride PET/CT Bone Scans. http://interactive.snm.org/docs/Procedure_Outline_NaF_PETV1.0.pdf. Accessed 15 July 2010.

Stein PD, Woodard PK, Weg JG, et al. Diagnostic pathways in acute pulmonary embolism: recommendations of the PIOPED II investigators. Radiology. 2007;242:15–21.

U.S. Environmental Protection Agency. Radiation Glossary. http://www.epa.gov/rpdweb00/rert/radfacts.html. Accessed 23 Sept 2010.

U.S. NRC. Procedures for receiving and opening packages. http://www.nrc.gov/reading-rm/doccollections/cfr/part020/part020-1906.html. Accessed 3 Sept 2010.

Vallabhajosula S, Killeen R, Osborne J. Altered biodistribution of radiopharmaceuticals: role of radiochemical/pharmaceutical purity, physiological, and pharmacologic factors. Semin Nucl Med. 2010;40:220–41.

Vitola J, Delbeke D. Nuclear cardiology and correlative imaging. New York, NY: Springer; 2004.

Wahl RL. Principles and practice of PET and PET/CT. 2nd ed. Philadelphia, PA: Lippincott and Wilkins; 2009.

Wikipedia. International System of Units. http://en.wikipedia.org/wiki/International_System_of_Units. Accessed 19 June 2010

Zanzonico P. Routine quality control of clinical nuclear medicine instrumentation: a brief review. J Nucl Med. 2008;49:1114–31.

Zaret BL, Beller GA. Clinical nuclear cardiology: state of the art and future directions. 3rd ed. Philadelphia, PA: Mosby; 2005.

Ziessman H. Interventions used with cholescintigraphy for the diagnosis of hepatobiliary disease. Semin Nucl Med. 2009;39:174–85.

Zuckier LS, Kolano J. Radionuclide studies in the determination of brain death: criteria, concepts, and controversies. Semin Nucl Med. 2008;38:262–73.

Chapter 4
Practice Test #3: Difficulty Level – Hard*

Questions

1. Pyuria is a common finding in renal disease and is defined as the presence of:
   (A) White cells in the urine
   (B) Blood in the urine
   (C) Casts in the urine
   (D) Protein in the urine

2. Gated single photon emission computed tomography myocardial perfusion imaging (SPECT MPI) can evaluate regional wall motion and ventricular volumes. Benefit of the combined assessment of myocardial perfusion and function relate to all of the following EXCEPT:
   (A) Help to differentiate attenuation artifacts from ischemia
   (B) Aid to identify patients with multivessel coronary artery disease
   (C) Assist in diagnosing arrhythmias
   (D) Provide prognostic value

3. Bilinear scaling methods employed in combined positron emission tomography/computed tomography (PET/CT) scanners software are used to:
   (A) Convert CT image values to PET attenuation coefficients
   (B) Correct image misregistration
   (C) Improve counting statistics of the PET acquisition
   (D) Adjust positional mismatches

---

*Answers to Test #3 begin on page 212.

A. Moniuszko and D. Patel, *Nuclear Medicine Technology Study Guide: A Technologist's Review for Passing Board Exams*, DOI 10.1007/978-1-4419-9362-5_4, © Springer Science+Business Media, LLC 2011

4. A patient referred for Meckel's diverticulum imaging received Cimetidine orally every 6 h for 1 day before the diagnostic imaging commenced. Cimetidine was given in what purpose?

(A) To inhibit secretion of pertechnetate into the bowel
(B) To stimulate pertechnetate accumulation in gastric mucosa
(C) To prevent pertechnetate accumulation in the thyroid
(D) To stop gastrointestinal bleeding

5. Figure 4.1 presents the schematic drawing of the normal heart conduction system. The label "D" represents:

(A) The left bundle branch
(B) The right bundle branch
(C) The sinoatrial node
(D) The atrioventricular node

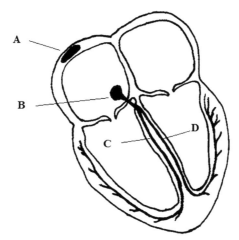

Fig. 4.1 Schematic drawing of normal heart conduction system (*Illustration by Sabina Moniuszko*)

6. Acute radiation syndrome (ARS) is defined as an acute illness caused by irradiation of the entire body (or most of the body) by a high dose of radiation in a very short period of time. What is the other requirement for the valid ARS diagnosis?

(A) The radiation must be penetrating
(B) The dose must be internal
(C) Radiation injuries must involve hands
(D) Patient must recover in 6 months

7. For Food and Drug Administration (FDA) approved positron emitting radio-pharmaceuticals the average range of positrons in human tissue is about:

   (A) 0.6–4 mm
   (B) 4–5 mm
   (C) 5–10 mm
   (D) >1 cm

8. The conventional transverse cross section is presented as a physician's view when at the bedside facing a recumbent patient from the patient's right side and looking up from below. On the transverse cross section image:

   (A) The anterior surface is down and the right side is on the left
   (B) The anterior surface is up and the right side is on the right
   (C) The anterior surface is up and the right side is on the left
   (D) The anterior surface is down and the right side is on the right

9. Background counts obtained by a well counter are as follows: 89, 103, 110, 117, and 125. What is the standard deviation of the obtained values from this WC?

   (A) 18
   (B) 17
   (C) 16
   (D) 14

10. Pentetreotide, a diethylene triamine pentaacetic acid (DTPA) conjugate of octreotide, synthetic analogue of natural somatostatin, localizes in various primary and metastatic neuroendocrine tumors bearing somatostatin receptor. All of the following tumors can be successfully diagnosed with In-111 Octreoscan EXCEPT:

    (A) Carcinoids
    (B) Gastrinomas
    (C) Sarcomas
    (D) Insulinomas

11. In the sitting and standing positions, blood flow per unit lung volume physiologically prevails in the lower lung lobes. In the patients with left heart disease, perfusion is redistributed with the upper/lower ratio:

    (A) Greater than 1.0
    (B) Equal to 1.0
    (C) Less than 1.0
    (D) Unchanged

12. Metaiodobenzylguanidine structurally resembles noradrenaline and when
    labeled with I-123, it is used in the detection of primary or metastatic pheo-
    chromocytoma or neuroblastoma. According to the package insert GE
    Healthcare AdreView™ Iobenguane I-123 injection, which of the following
    group of medications should be reviewed for potentially being withdrawn
    prior to imaging?
    (A) Antibiotics
    (B) Anticoagulants
    (C) Antihypertensives
    (D) Antiepileptics

13. If one orients the ring of left ventricle myocardial activity on myocardial perfu-
    sion imaging (MPI), as it were a clock, the right coronary artery is the primary
    vessel in the area:
    (A) 7–10 o'clock
    (B) 10–1 o'clock
    (C) 1–5 o'clock
    (D) 5–7 o'clock

14. Which of the following answers correctly identifies sequencing of imaging
    during hepatobiliary scintigraphy?
    (A) Gallbladder ejection fraction, perfusion, parenchymal uptake
    (B) Parenchymal uptake, perfusion, gallbladder ejection fraction
    (C) Perfusion, gallbladder ejection fraction, parenchymal uptake
    (D) Perfusion, parenchymal uptake, gallbladder ejection fraction

15. Figure 4.2 presents the images obtained during 2 h hepatobiliary scintig-
    raphy after intravenous injection of 6.0 mCi of Tc-99m Choletec. Which
    of the following statements is most consistent with the findings from the
    scan?
    (A) Normal hepatobiliary scan
    (B) Sphincter of Oddi obstruction
    (C) Cystic duct obstruction
    (D) Liver cirrhosis

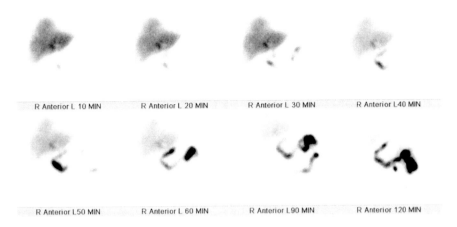

R Anterior L 10 MIN   R Anterior L 20 MIN   R Anterior L 30 MIN   R Anterior L40 MIN

R Anterior L50 MIN   R Anterior L 60 MIN   R Anterior L90 MIN   R Anterior 120 MIN

Fig. 4.2 Hepatobiliary scintigraphy

16. Radon is responsible for the majority of the mean public exposure to ionizing radiation and it is often the single largest contributor to an individual's background radiation dose. Which of the following statements regarding radon and radon exposure is FALSE?

    (A) It varies from location to location
    (B) Radon is formed as part of the normal radioactive decay chain of uranium
    (C) Radon is the most frequent cause of lung cancer
    (D) Radon test kits are commercially available

17. An electron, stripped from an atom as a charged particle, passes through matter that has enough kinetic energy to cause subsequent ionization at a distant site is called:

    (A) Compton electron
    (B) X-ray
    (C) Delta ray
    (D) Gamma ray

18. Which of the following is an example of a "rigid" body organ?

    (A) Heart
    (B) Liver
    (C) Brain
    (D) Lung

19. How many dpm (disintegrations per minute) are produced by source that is reading 4,850 cpm (counts per minute) in well counter? Well-counter efficiency is 56% and background counts are 150 cpm.
    (A) 4,149 dpm
    (B) 6,208 dpm
    (C) 7,632 dpm
    (D) 8,393 dpm

20. Ga-67 citrate accumulates as an iron analogue through binding to circulating transferrin and 10–25% of the radionuclide is excreted via the kidneys during the first 24 h. After 24 h the principal route of excretion is:
    (A) Saliva
    (B) Sweat
    (C) Hepatobiliary
    (D) Skin

21. The results of the study, known as INTERSTROKE, identified nine modifiable risk factors for stroke and accounting for 90% of disease. According to the study the strongest risk factor for stroke was:
    (A) Alcohol intake
    (B) Hypertension
    (C) Cigarette smoking
    (D) Obesity

22. Sentinel lymph node biopsy is a multidisciplinary technique in which nuclear medicine performs preoperative lymphoscintigraphy. Which method is utilized by surgeons to identify the sentinel node?
    (A) Gamma probe and/or blue dye
    (B) Gamma-camera and/or blue dye
    (C) Gamma probe and/or red dye
    (D) Gamma-camera and/or red dye

23. The term "partial volume effect" is caused by the limited resolution of PET scanners and refers to phenomenon that make intensity values in images differ from what they ideally should be. The "hot" spot smaller than twice the resolution of the scanner will have total counts preserved and will appear:
    (A) Larger with a higher activity concentration
    (B) Larger with a lower activity concentration
    (C) Smaller with a higher activity concentration
    (D) Smaller with a lower activity concentration

24. Symmetrically increased uptake of the radiotracer in the cortices ("tram lines") observed on the bone scintigraphy can be present in patients diagnosed with:
    (A) Hypertrophic pulmonary osteoarthropathy
    (B) Osteogenesis imperfecta
    (C) Paget's disease
    (D) Osteomyelosclerosis

25. Figure 4.3 presents the diagrams of end-systolic (dashed line) and end-diastolic (solid line) shape of left ventricle cineangiogram. The drawing (a) represents normal left ventricle wall motion. What left ventricle abnormality corresponds to the drawing (b)?
    (A) Hypokinetic left ventricle
    (B) Hyperkinetic left ventricle
    (C) Akinetic left ventricle
    (D) Dyskinetic left ventricle

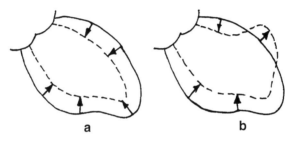

Fig. 4.3 End-systolic (dashed line) and end-diastolic (solid line) shape of left ventricle cineangiogram (*Illustration by Sabina Moniuszko*)

26. Estimates of absorbed organ doses, as well as effective doses from nuclear medicine procedures, are available from all of the following sources EXCEPT:
    (A) Patient information booklets
    (B) Nuclear medicine textbooks
    (C) Food and Drug Administration-required inserts
    (D) Society of Nuclear Medicine procedure guidelines

27. A plot of activity of decay vs. time on semilogarithmic paper will generate:
    (A) A parabola
    (B) A hyperbola
    (C) A sinusoidal wave
    (D) A straight line

28. Windowing or contrast enhancement is an example of a very common form of digital processing of images using:
    (A) Digital-to-analog converter (DAC)
    (B) Lookup table (LUT)
    (C) Analog-to-digital converter (ADC)
    (D) Standardized uptake value (SUV)

29. If a long-lived source produces 56,890 counts per minute (cpm), what is the expectable range of values within three standard deviations or at 99% confidence level?
    (A) Between 56,794 and 56,989 cpm
    (B) Between 56,421 and 57,506 cpm
    (C) Between 56,174 and 57,606 cpm
    (D) Between 56,000 and 57,810 cpm

30. A round or ovoid congenital bony defect that results from incomplete fusion of the sternal ossification centers and presented on a bone scan as a photopenic, well-delineated rounded area is called:
    (A) Sternal angle
    (B) Sternal notch
    (C) Sternal foramina
    (D) Sternal dehiscence.

31. After intravenous catheter removal, gauze is placed over the site and gentle pressure is applied for 2–3 min. This time should be extended for patients taking:
    (A) Digoxin
    (B) Clopidogrel
    (C) Captopril
    (D) Atenolol

32. Flow images acquired during brain death scintigraphy are assessed for blood flow to the brain. Which view is preferred when the brain flow study is performed?
    (A) Anterior
    (B) Posterior
    (C) Right or left lateral
    (D) Anterior or posterior oblique

33. The correlation between the number of counts and display intensity is commonly linear which provides uniform shading between all counts intensities. An exponential relationship between the number of counts and display intensity:

    (A) Suppresses low counts
    (B) Enhances high count
    (C) Enhances low counts
    (D) Compresses the number of shades in the high pixel values

34. In the majority of patients active bleeding can be detected by angiography if the rate of bleeding is in excess of:

    (A) 0.1 ml/min
    (B) 0.3 ml/min
    (C) 0.5 ml/min
    (D) 1 ml/min

35. Images presented in Fig. 4.4 are acquired during liver–spleen scintigraphy after intravenous administration of 6.1 mCi of Tc-99m sulfur colloid. Which view is missing on the presented display?

    (A) Posterior marker
    (B) Flow
    (C) Blood pool
    (D) RPO

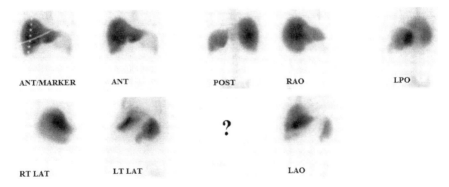

Fig. 4.4 Liver-spleen scintigraphy

36. Collective dosage to the US population from nuclear medicine procedures includes not only the dose to the patient but also doses to members of the public from other nuclear medicine patients. For most diagnostic studies, the dose rate at 1 m from the patient immediately after injection is about:

    (A) 0.5–2.0 Gy/h
    (B) 2–20 Gy/h
    (C) 20–100 Gy/h
    (D) 100–300 Gy/h

37. I-123 and I-131 are radioactive isotopes of iodine used for diagnostic purposes in nuclear medicine. All of the following statements describing their properties are true EXCEPT:
    (A) I-131 has longer half-life than I-123
    (B) I-123 is reactor and I-131 is cyclotron produced
    (C) I-123 is a pure gamma and I-131 is a gamma and beta emitter
    (D) I-123 has greater photon flux than I-131

38. Positron emission tomography (PET) blank scans are performed daily and represent the sensitivity response of the transmission source without any atten-uating material present in the gantry. Acquired data are applied for:
    (A) SUV calculation
    (B) Image reconstruction
    (C) Energy window calibrations
    (D) Attenuation correction

39. A vial of Ga-67 produces exposure rate of 25 mR/h. How many half-value lay-ers (HVLs) and thickness of lead will reduce the exposure rate to less than 1 mR/h? Half-value layer (HVL) for Ga-67 is 0.10 cm.
    (A) 1 HVLs and 0.8 cm
    (B) 2 HVLs and 0.7 cm
    (C) 4 HVLs and 0.6 cm
    (D) 5 HVLs and 0.5 cm

40. Blood within the gut lumen stimulates strong peristaltic action resulting in the spread of the blood from the site of bleeding:
    (A) Antegrade
    (B) Retrograde
    (C) Posteriograde
    (D) Antegrade and retrograde

41. The process of mineral exchange and new bone formation, by which new bone gradually replaces old bone is called bone:
    (A) Activation
    (B) Acquisition
    (C) Accretion
    (D) Avulsion

42. All of the following account for the difficulties of detection and localization of bleeding in small bowel on gastrointestinal bleeding scintigraphy EXCEPT:
    (A) Small bowel is more prone to overlap with vascular structures
    (B) Small bowel is more variable in location
    (C) Small bowel has a tendency for a greater anterograde and retrograde peristalsis
    (D) Small bowel transit time is slower

43. Well-counter calibration data of a positron emission tomography (PET) scanner are applied for:

(A) Standardized uptake value (SUV) calculation
(B) Image reconstruction
(C) Energy window calibrations
(D) Attenuation correction

44. According to the current procedure guideline of the Society of Nuclear Medicine, the use of delayed imaging when performing gastrointestinal bleeding scintigraphy with Tc-99m tagged red blood cells is:

(A) Optional
(B) Recommended
(C) Obligatory
(D) Not indicated

45. Figure 4.5 presents the flow images obtained during gastrointestinal bleeding scintigraphy with Tc-99m-labeled red blood cells. Which of the following statements is most consistent with the findings from the scan?

(A) Normal scan
(B) Active bleeding – ascending colon
(C) Active bleeding – descending colon
(D) Liver hemangioma

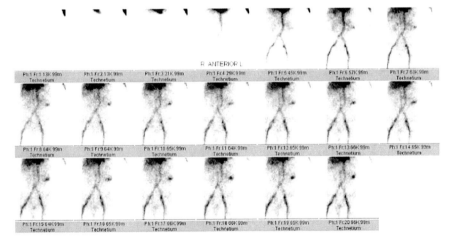

Fig. 4.5 Gastrointestinal bleeding scintigraphy

46. Data on the number of nuclear medicine examinations performed between 1972 and 2005 indicate the most dramatic increase occurred in cardiac imaging procedures. Cardiac studies are relatively high-dose procedures and account for more than:

    (A) 45% of the effective dose to the patient population
    (B) 60% of the effective dose to the patient population
    (C) 85% of the effective dose to the patient population
    (D) 95% of the effective dose to the patient population

47. Before the administration of a radiopharmaceutical into a human subject, several quality control tests need to be performed. The biological tests establish the radiopharmaceutical:

    (A) Apyrogenicity
    (B) Purity
    (C) Chemistry
    (D) Integrity

48. F-18 is a cyclotron-produced radioisotope with a half-life approximately of:

    (A) 11 min
    (B) 101 min
    (C) 110 min
    (D) 119 min

49. The radiopharmacy has 423 mCi of I-131 calibrated on Monday at 10:00 A.M. and three orders for I-131 therapy doses throughout the week. If the therapy doses are needed as described below, how much activity will be remaining after all three doses are withdrawn? ($T\frac{1}{2}$ of I-131 is 8 days)

    Tuesday 80 mCi at 10:00 A.M.
    Thursday 110 mCi at 10:00 A.M.
    Friday 130 mCi at 10:00 A.M.
    (A) 7 mCi
    (B) 10 mCi
    (C) 12 mCi
    (D) 14 mCi

50. Metastatic calcification is described as calcium deposition in normal tissues due to hypercalcemia and it may be seen in patients diagnosed with:

    (A) Hyperparathyroidism
    (B) Vitamin C-related disorders
    (C) Hepatosplenomegaly
    (D) Osteomyelitis

51. The outer layer of the cerebral hemispheres is called the cerebral cortex and is composed of:
    (A) White matter
    (B) Pia mater
    (C) Gray matter
    (D) Dura mater

52. Which of the following tumors is most likely to be associated with increased Tc-99m methylene diphosphonate (MDP) uptake?
    (A) Mucinous adenocarcinoma
    (B) Hemangioma
    (C) Benign cyst
    (D) Colon carcinoma

53. The Hounsfield unit or CT (computed tomography) number relates to the composition and nature of the tissue imaged and is used to represent the density of tissue. An arbitrarily assigned number to water is equal to 0 and the CT number assigned to air is equal to:
    (A) −1,000
    (B) −100
    (C) 100
    (D) 1,000

54. Images obtained shortly after injection of leukocytes labeled with In-111 or Tc-99m are characterized by intense pulmonary activity that clears and approaches background level by:
    (A) 0.5 h after injection
    (B) 1 h after injection
    (C) 2 h after injection
    (D) 4 h after injection

55. Figure 4.6 displays images acquired during 32 frames multigated acquisition (MUGA) scan. On the presented display the end diastole image is labeled:
    (A) d
    (B) c
    (C) b
    (D) a

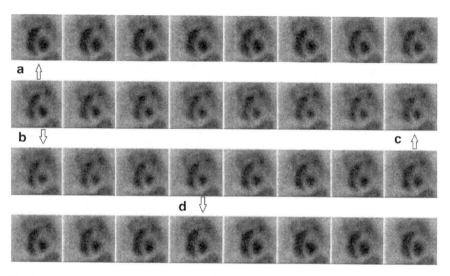

Fig. 4.6 Multi gated acquisition (MUGA) scan

56. The combined positron emission tomography/computed tomography (PET/CT) scans have an effective dose to the patients in the range of:
    (A) 0.5–20 mSv
    (B) 20–40 mSv
    (C) 40–80 mSv
    (D) 80–160 mSv

57. The contamination of other radioisotopes of iodine depends on the nuclear reaction used for the production of I-123 in a cyclotron. The two major radionuclide impurities in I-123 sodium iodide capsules are:
    (A) I-124 and I-131
    (B) I-124 and I-125
    (C) I-125 and I-131
    (D) I-126 and I-131

58. Filtered backprojection (FBP) and iterative reconstruction (IR) are two common reconstructions techniques employed in nuclear medicine. Which of the following statements describing their properties is FALSE?
    (A) FBP in low counts SPECT amplifies noise
    (B) FBP is unable to correct for scatter
    (C) IR requires higher counts density
    (D) IR is computationally demanding

59. Ga-67 is excreted from the body with two different biological half-lives. A small fraction of Ga-67 is excreted with a biological half-life of 30 h and the majority of the Ga-67 is excreted with a biological half-life of 25 days. What are the two effective half-lives of Ga-67?
   (A) 12 h and 22 days
   (B) 20 h and 13 days
   (C) 22 h and 3 days
   (D) 32 h and 3 days

60. Ga-67 citrate and Tc-99m or In-111-labeled leukocyte imaging are well-established procedures for diagnosing a variety of inflammatory and infectious conditions. Normally healing surgical incisions will concentrate:
   (A) In-111-labeled leukocytes
   (B) Tc-99m-labeled leukocytes
   (C) Ga-67 citrate
   (D) Tl-201 citrate

61. A 56-year-old man with chest pain, atrial fibrillation, and an abnormal myocardial perfusion imaging treadmill stress test underwent a procedure frequently abbreviated as a percutaneous transluminal coronary angioplasty (PTCA). Performed PTCA procedure is also called:
   (A) Ablation for atrial fibrillation
   (B) Angioplasty
   (C) Calcium scoring
   (D) Bypass surgery

62. Gallbladder ejection fraction creates objective and quantitative measure of:
   (A) Bile production
   (B) Gallbladder function
   (C) Hepatic perfusion
   (D) Parenchymal arrangement

63. All of the following statements describing new imaging technologies using cadmium–zinc–telluride (CZT) detectors when compared with the parallel collimated Anger cameras are true EXCEPT:
   (A) New imaging technologies have sensitivities of 2.2–4.7 while Anger cameras 0.5–0.7 kcps
   (B) CZT-based SPECT cameras have Tc-99m energy resolution 9–10% vs. 5.7% of Anger's
   (C) CZT-based SPECT cameras have spatial resolution 4–5 mm vs. 9–10 mm of Anger's
   (D) CZT-based high-quality images can be acquired with greatly reduced injected dose

64. Which of the following will be helpful to differentiate rectal from bladder activity when performing Tc-99m Labeled RBC's bleeding scan?
   (A) Delay imaging
   (B) Dynamic imaging
   (C) Lateral views
   (D) Image of the bed pan

65. Images presented in Fig. 4.7 were obtained during routine bone scintigraphy from two different patients. Upper row images belong to the patient A and lower row images belong to the patient B. Which of the following statements is most consistent with the findings from these scans?
   (A) Both patients have normal scans
   (B) Patient B has rib fractures, patient A has bone metastases
   (C) Patient A has rib fractures, patient B has bone metastases
   (D) Both patients have bone metastases

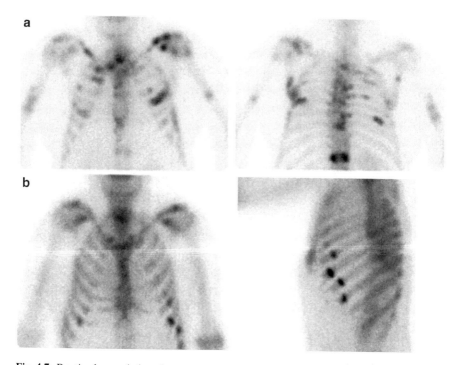

Fig. 4.7 Routine bone scintigraphy

66. The effective dose expressed in units of milisiverts (mSv) is a wide-ranging approximation of the risk of biologic injury from a partial exposure to ionizing radiation that allows comparisons between all of the following EXCEPT:

    (A) Different imaging protocols
    (B) Different types of radiological examinations
    (C) Different natural or man-made sources of radiation
    (D) Different patients

67. The radiochemical purity of a radiopharmaceutical can be tested with all of the following EXCEPT:

    (A) Gel electrophoresis
    (B) Instant thin layer chromatography
    (C) Ion exchange
    (D) Liquid scintillation counter

68. The system for display of medical images on computer workstations for preliminary diagnosis and for permanent archiving of digital images is commonly referred and abbreviated as:

    (A) DIACOM
    (B) PACS
    (C) LAN
    (D) CPU

69. How many microcuries (μCi) is 6.3 gigabecquerels (GBq)?

    (A) 171 μCi
    (B) 1,701 μCi
    (C) 170,100 μCi
    (D) 17,01,000 μCi

70. The concentration of glucose-6-phosphatase, an enzyme mediating dephosphorylation of FDG-6-phosphate, is low in most tumors EXCEPT:

    (A) Lung adenocarcinoma
    (B) Hepatocellular carcinoma
    (C) Hodgkin lymphoma
    (D) Ductal carcinoma

71. The most common type of ectopic tissue in Meckel's diverticulum is:

    (A) Gastric mucosa
    (B) Duodenal mucosa
    (C) Intestinal mucosa
    (D) Esophageal mucosa

72. All of the following cellular mechanisms are responsible for malignant cells increased F-18 fluorodeoxyglucose accumulation EXCEPT:
    (A) Increased membrane transporters
    (B) Increased intracellular hexokinase
    (C) Low glucose-6-phosphatase
    (D) Low mitotic rate

73. A sequence of independent, identically distributed pulses arriving at random times, and detected by the scintillation detector is called:
    (A) White noise
    (B) Scatter
    (C) Background
    (D) Attenuation

74. The elevated serum glucose level at the time of fluorodeoxyglucose (FDG) administration may decrease the sensitivity of the FDG-PET study. Althoguh intravenous bolus of insulin may effectively lower the serum glucose level, however induced hyperinsulinemia will:
    (A) Shunt glucose to skeletal and cardiac muscles
    (B) Induce hyperglycemia
    (C) Increase blood pressure
    (D) Decrease heart rate

75. Image presented in Fig. 4.8 labeled as image (D) – left lateral view of the chest – was acquired during routine bone scintigraphy from the patient:
    (A) C
    (B) A
    (C) B
    (D) A, B, and C

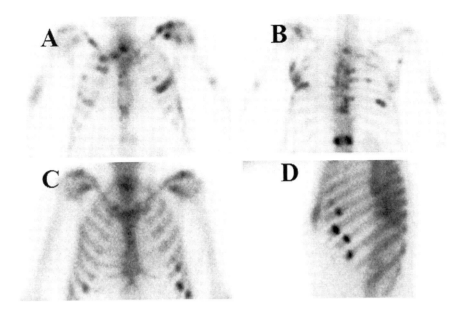

Fig. 4.8 Routine bone scintigraphy

76. All breastfeeding women undergoing I-131 therapy should be asked to stop breastfeeding and therapy is delayed until lactation ceases. According to the Society of Nuclear Medicine (SNM) procedure guidelines, the patient may resume breastfeeding:
    (A) With the birth of another child
    (B) Never
    (C) After 6 months
    (D) After 3 months

77. Which of the following radionuclides has the highest kinetic energy of the positron?
    (A) C-11
    (B) F-18
    (C) Rb-82
    (D) N-13

78. All of the following methods can be used to estimate the spatial resolution of gamma-camera detectors EXCEPT:
    (A) Point spread function
    (B) Bar patterns
    (C) High counts flood
    (D) Line spread function

79. A Tc-99m mebrofenin kit was prepared at 8:00 A.M. At the time of preparation,
    the kit contained 35.7 mCi of Tc-99m in 4 ml. What is the concentration of
    Tc-99m in the mebrofenin kit at 3:30 P.M. on the same day?
    (A) 3.8 mCi/ml
    (B) 5.3 mCi/ml
    (C) 8.9 mCi/ml
    (D) 21.4 mCi/ml

80. Which of the following statements comparing normal findings on SPECT and
    PET/CT bone imaging is correct?
    (A) PET/CT has higher resolution and visualized physiologic variability is
        more prominent
    (B) PET/CT has higher resolution and visualized physiologic variability is
        less prominent
    (C) PET/CT has lower resolution and visualized physiologic variability is
        more prominent
    (D) There is no difference in visualized physiologic variability

81. The PR interval is measured from the beginning of the P wave to the first part
    of the QRS complex and its length:
    (A) Does not change with heart rate
    (B) Is longer at faster heart rates
    (C) Is shorter at lower heart rates
    (D) Is longer with an increase in vagal inputs

82. The severity of the breast attenuation artifact on myocardial perfusion
    scintigraphy is:
    (A) Directly proportional to the breast size
    (B) Directly proportional to chest circumference
    (C) Varies with the density of the breast
    (D) Varies with the patient weight

83. The postprocessing attenuation technique that applies a constant attenuation
    coefficient and requires prior knowledge of the edge of the object (body
    boundaries) is called:
    (A) Backprojection attenuation correction
    (B) Transmission-based attenuation correction
    (C) Chang attenuation correction
    (D) Iterative attenuation correction

84. Breast attenuation and lateral chest-wall fat attenuation in myocardial perfusion scintigraphy can produce areas of markedly decreased count density. The attenuation artifact caused by the lateral chest-wall fat usually:

    (A) Is more diffuse than breast attenuation artifact
    (B) Is limited to the inferior wall
    (C) Is limited to the anterior wall
    (D) Is more prominent on the resting images

85. Figure 4.9 presents reconstruction reoriented SPECT data of the patient's heart and created short axis slices. On the diagram the label "D" corresponds to the:

    (A) Anterior wall
    (B) Septal wall
    (C) Inferior wall
    (D) Lateral wall

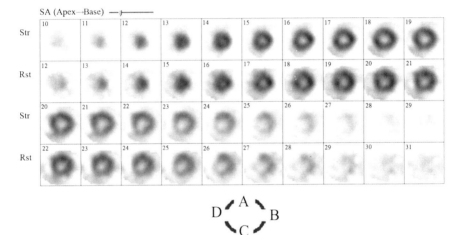

Fig. 4.9 Reconstruction reoriented SPECT data

86. Indirect effect of radiation exposure in body tissues is primarily mediated by:

    (A) Radiolytic decomposition of water in a cell
    (B) Deoxyribonucleic acid (DNA) damage
    (C) Mitochondrial death
    (D) Cell membrane lysis

87. Which of the following radionuclides used in PET imaging produces the highest resolution images?

    (A) C-11
    (B) F-18
    (C) Rb-82
    (D) N-13

88. Segmentation, scaling, or a hybrid technique, are commonly used methods to:
    (A) Convert the CT image into an attenuation map
    (B) Convert an attenuation map into Hounsfield units
    (C) Calculate standardized uptake value (SUV)
    (D) Calculate Chang attenuation coefficient

89. Counts listed below were obtained from the patient's neck and thigh 24 h after ingestion of 300 μCi I-123 capsule. What is the percentage of thyroid uptake at 24 h?

    300 μCi I-123 capsules –345,890 cpm Background –111 cpm
    Thyroid   –80,123 cpm   Thigh   –5,324 cpm

    24 h I-123 decay factor – 0.284

    (A) 81%
    (B) 76%
    (C) 64%
    (D) 55%

90. The presence of interventricular septal flattening on gated SPECT studies correlates with:
    (A) Right ventricle (RV) overload
    (B) Left ventricle (LV) overload
    (C) Transient ischemic dilation (TID)
    (D) Myocardial ischemia

91. The QRS complex represents the time for ventricular depolarization and is characterized by all of the following EXCEPT:
    (A) An entirely negative QRS complex is called a QS wave
    (B) The negative deflection following the R wave is the S wave
    (C) The entire QRS duration normally lasts for 0.06–0.10 s
    (D) The QRS duration is influenced by heart rate

92. Matching SPECT prone tomographic myocardial perfusion imaging is recommended for more accurate assessment of the right coronary artery (RCA) stenosis. In the prone position:
    (A) There is more upward creep
    (B) There is more motion of the anterior chest
    (C) The heart shifts posteriorly
    (D) The diaphragm is pushed down

93. All of the following statements describing the Geiger–Mueller (G-M) counter are true EXCEPT:
    (A) G-M provides a high electron amplification factor
    (B) Geiger counters are calibrated in counting rates (cpm)
    (C) Geiger counters well suited for low-level surveys
    (D) Amplitude of the signal pulses is dependent on the energy of the incoming radiation

94. Discovered reversible perfusion defects in patients with left bundle branch block (LBBB) who underwent treadmill myocardial perfusion studies can mimic stress-induced ischemia in myocardial:
    (A) Septum
    (B) Inferior wall
    (C) Anterior wall
    (D) Apex

95. Figure 4.10 presents the schematic diagram of the hepatobiliary tract. What part of the hepatobiliary tree represents label "a"?
    (A) Sphincter of Oddi
    (B) Cystic duct
    (C) Common bile duct
    (D) Common hepatic duct

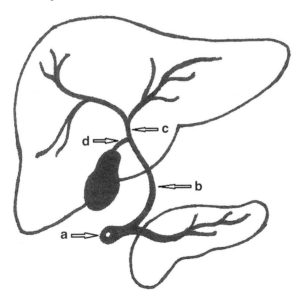

Fig. 4.10 Schematic diagram of the hepatobiliary tract (*Illustration by Sabina Moniuszko*)

96. The average person in the USA receives an effective dose from naturally occurring radioactive materials and cosmic radiation:
    (A) Dose of about 1 mSv per year
    (B) Dose of about 2 mSv per year
    (C) Dose of about 3 mSv per year
    (D) Dose of about 5 mSv per year

97. Astatine-211, bismuth-212, and radium-223 are examples of:
    (A) Alpha-particle emitters
    (B) Beta-particle emitters
    (C) Alpha- and beta-particle emitters
    (D) Pure gamma emitters

98. For transportation purposes, radioactive material is defined as any material which has a specific activity greater than:
    (A) 0.001 microcurie/g
    (B) 0.002 microcurie/g
    (C) 0.004 microcurie/g
    (D) 0.006 microcurie/g

99. A Tc-99m Sestamibi vial contains 68 mCi in 3.0 ml at 10:00 A.M. What volume volume should be drawn into syringe at 13:00, if a 24 mCi Sestamibi dose is needed?
    (A) 1.5 ml
    (B) 2.1 mCi
    (C) 2.7 ml
    (D) 3.2 ml

100. The relatively low resolution of nuclear cardiology images may make visualization of small objects difficult. Quantitative error elicited by this phenomenon is called:
    (A) Blurring effect
    (B) Zooming effect
    (C) Partial volume effect
    (D) Count drop-of effect

101. A form of cell death in which a programmed sequence of events leads to the elimination of cells without releasing harmful substances into the surrounding area is called:
    (A) Phagocytosis
    (B) Pinocytosis
    (C) Apoptosis
    (D) Endocytosis

102. The 17-segment model for semiquantitative analysis of perfusion defects has become the preferred nomenclature. How many basal segments are in this representation?
    (A) 4
    (B) 5
    (C) 6
    (D) 7

103. To verify that the survey meter has not been contaminated during the preceding operation, the technologist should check:
    (A) The background counting rate
    (B) The survey meter battery
    (C) The survey meter constancy of response
    (D) The survey meter accuracy of response

104. How much of the administered activity will remain in the blood 3 hrs after injection of Tc99m MDP?
    (A) 3%
    (B) 13%
    (C) 23%
    (D) 33%

105. Figure 4.11 presents the dynamic, flow images obtained during what type of nuclear medicine study?
    (A) 3-Phase bone scintigraphy
    (B) Brain death scintigraphy
    (C) Renal scintigraphy with Lasix
    (D) Ventriculoperitoneal shunt patency scintigraphy

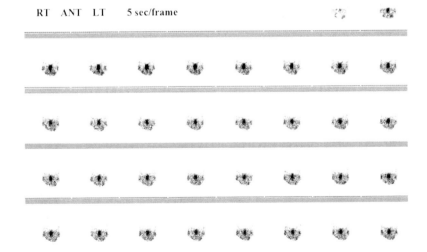

RT ANT LT   5 sec/frame

Fig. 4.11 Dynamic images

106. Radiation exposure in younger patients results in a greater lifetime risk of potential radiation-induced cancer than in older patients. Calculated lifetime risk of cancer from a specific radiologic, examination in a 20-year-old woman, when comparing with a 50-year-old man is:
    (A) Two times greater
    (B) Three times greater
    (C) Four times greater
    (D) Five times greater

107. All of the following are examples of generators yielding positron-emitting daughter radionuclides EXCEPT:
    (A) Strontium-82
    (B) Germanium-68
    (C) Oxygen-15
    (D) Xenon-122

108. All of the following long-lived sources can be used in nuclear medicine departments for instrumentation quality control procedures EXCEPT:
    (A) Cs-137
    (B) Ba-133
    (C) Co-60
    (D) Ge-68

109. A patient is scheduled to have a Rb-82 PET scan for myocardial infarction at 9:30 A.M. If 30 mCi of a Rb-82 dose is needed at 9:30 A.M., how many millicuries (mCi) should be withdrawn in the syringe at 9:27 A.M. on the same day? (Precalibration factor is 5.3)
    (A) 59 mCi
    (B) 118 mCi
    (C) 159 mCi
    (D) 189 mCi

110. Transient ischemic dilation (TID) is defined as an increase in left ventricle (LV) size at stress compared to rest and its presence correlates with all of the following EXCEPT:
    (A) The extent and severity of coronary artery disease on coronary angiogram
    (B) The extent and severity of the perfusion abnormalities
    (C) The degree and extent of ST depression on electrocardiogram (ECG)
    (D) The incidence and extent of arrhythmias on electrocardiogram (ECG)

111. The tricuspid valve separates:
    (A) The left atrium from the left ventricle
    (B) The right atrium from the right ventricle
    (C) The left ventricle from the aorta
    (D) The right ventricle from the pulmonary artery

112. Prospective investigation of pulmonary embolism diagnosis (PIOPED II) was a multicenter trial conducted between 2000 and 2005 to determine the value of contrast-enhanced spiral computed tomography (spiral CT) for the diagnosis of acute pulmonary embolism (PE). Which two major widely used technologies were evaluated in PIOPED I trial?
    (A) Magnetic resonance venography and spiral CT
    (B) Ventilation–perfusion scanning and pulmonary angiography
    (C) Magnetic resonance angiography and ventilation–perfusion scanning
    (D) Ventilation–perfusion scanning and spiral CT

113. Scintillation well counters have high intrinsic and geometric efficiencies and can reliably count activities up to approximately:
    (A) 0.37 kBq
    (B) 3.7 kBq
    (C) 37 kBq
    (D) 370 kBq

114. The presence of the heart in the right hemithorax, with the cardiac apex directed to the right is called:
    (A) Cardioversion
    (B) Dextrocardia
    (C) Mesocardia
    (D) Isolated levocardia

115. The myocardial perfusion can be estimated by analyzing bull's-eye display of the resting perfusion-labeled "A" and the stress perfusion-labeled "B." Images presented in Fig. 4.12 and displayed as a polar plot indicate the presence of a reversible defect in the area of myocardium supplied by:
    (A) Left circumflex artery (LCX)
    (B) Left anterior descending (LAD)
    (C) Left main artery (LMA)
    (D) Right coronary artery (RCA)

a   b

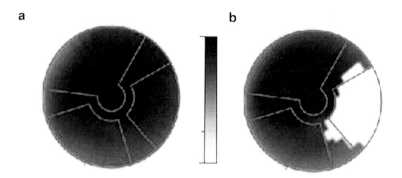

Fig. 4.12 Bull's-eye display of the resting and the stress myocardial perfusion

116. When reviewing federal guidelines, states that intend to sign an agreement with the Nuclear Regulatory Commission (NRC) may choose:
    (A) To be more restrictive than the Federal guidelines
    (B) To be less restrictive than the Federal guidelines
    (C) Do not follow the Federal guidelines
    (D) Review the Federal guidelines for future acceptance

117. The parent radionuclide of the generator produced positron-emitting Rubidium-82 is:
    (A) Strontium-82
    (B) Germanium-68
    (C) Xenon-122
    (D) Xenon-122

118. Which of the following tests is recommended for a 55 year old man with diabetes, low pretest probability for pulmonary embolism and positive D-dimer?
    (A) V/Q scan
    (B) CT scan with contrast
    (C) CT scan without contrast
    (D) PE excluded based on the information provided

119. How much minimum activity of Tc-99m is needed at 7:00 A.M. to prepare kits described below for the use on this day?
    MDP kit with 185 mCi at 8:00 A.M.
    MAA kit with 30 mCi at 10:00 A.M.
    Mebrofenin kit with 35 mCi at 12:00 P.M.
    (A) 312 mCi
    (B) 253 mCi
    (C) 248 mCi
    (D) 211 mCi

120. Flow imaging is an essential part of all of the following nuclear medicine procedures EXCEPT:

(A) 3-Phase bone scan for osteomyelitis diagnosis
(B) Tagged red blood cells (RBCs) for liver hemangioma imaging
(C) Tagged white blood cells for osteomyelitis diagnosis
(D) Tc-99m pertechnetate for brain death scintigraphy

121. The portion of the abdomen and pelvis which does not lie within the peritoneum is called the extraperitoneal space. Which of the following organ is situated extraperitoneally?

(A) Spleen
(B) Stomach
(C) Transverse colon
(D) Abdominal aorta

122. What is the usual range of a 24 hr radioiodine uptake in hyperthyroid patients diagnosed with subacute thyroiditis?

(A) ≤2%
(B) 2–20%
(C) 20–40%
(D) 40–80%

123. The basic procedure in the filtered backprojection technique is converting the frequency space into the spatial domain. This is known as:

(A) Filtering
(B) Volume rendering
(C) Inverse Fourier transform
(D) Convoluting

124. Based on their origin, non-Hodgkin's lymphomas are classified as either B-cell lymphomas or T-cell lymphomas. B-cells arise from reticuloendothelial elements in the prenatal liver and spleen and T-cells arise from:

(A) Thyroid
(B) Thymus
(C) Thalamus
(D) Tongue

125. Figure 4.13 displays four different I-123 thyroid scans images where image (a) demonstrates a normal thyroid gland. The findings from image (d) are most consistent with the clinical diagnosis of:

(A) Hypothyroidism
(B) Grave's disease
(C) Multinodular goiter
(D) Autonomously hyperfunctioning thyroid nodule

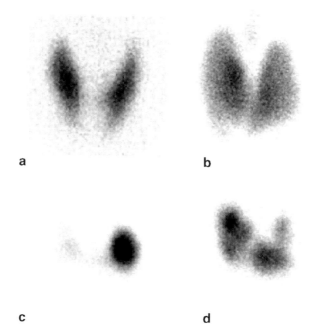

Fig. 4.13 I-123 thyroid scans images

126. Single-strand breaks (SSB), double-strand breaks (DSB), base damage, and multiple damaged sites (MDS), are radiation-induced biologic effects in the:
    (A) Ribonucleic acid (RNA)
    (B) Deoxyribonucleic acid (DNA)
    (C) Bone marrow
    (D) Liver

127. All of the following are examples of different types of photon interactions with matter EXCEPT:
    (A) Pair production
    (B) Photoelectric effect
    (C) Compton scatter
    (D) Iodination

128. Process of reconstruction of tomographic images by filtered backprojection (FBP) consists of four steps. Which one of the following is in the proper order for the FBP reconstruction?
    (A) Fourier transform, backprojection, inverse Fourier transform, filtering
    (B) Filtering, backprojection, Fourier transform, inverse Fourier transform
    (C) Backprojection, Fourier transform, filtering, inverse Fourier transform
    (D) Fourier transform, filtering, inverse Fourier transform, backprojection

129. A vial of Tc-99m methylene diphosphonate (MDP) contains 55 mCi in 3.5 ml at 9:00 A.M. on Monday. How much activity will be remaining in the vial after withdrawing 25 mCi at 1:00 P.M. the same day?
   (A) 10.5 mCi
   (B) 10 mCi
   (C) 2.5 mCi
   (D) 1.4 mCi

130. A chimeric monoclonal antibody against the protein CD-20 – primarily found on the surface of B-cells – is called:
   (A) Rituximab
   (B) Zevalin
   (C) Bexxar
   (D) Atacicept

131. There are 12 thoracic vertebrae. T 7 vertebra is located at the level of:
   (A) The highest point of the iliac crest
   (B) The medial part of the scapula
   (C) The inferior angle of the scapula
   (D) The posterior superior iliac spine

132. The relative coronary flow reserve (CFR), which provides a functional assessment of the severity of coronary stenosis is define as the ratio of:
   (A) Lung-to-heart uptake
   (B) RSS-to-SSS
   (C) Hyperemic flow velocity to the resting flow velocity
   (D) Hyperemic flow velocity in diseased artery to that of normal artery

133. All of the following agents have been used for scintigraphic pulmonary ventilation studies EXCEPT:
   (A) Tc-99m-labeled diethylenetriamine pentaacetic acid (DTPA) aerosol
   (B) Inert gas Kr-81m
   (C) Tc-99m-labeled Technegas
   (D) In-111-labeled diethylenetriamine pentaacetic acid (DTPA) aerosol

134. Which of the pharmacological interventions can be used in hepatobiliary scintigraphy to aid in the differential diagnosis of neonatal jaundice?
   (A) Morphine
   (B) Sincalide
   (C) Fatty meal
   (D) Phenobarbital

135. Figure 4.14. A 66 years old man with abdominal pain. Abdominal computerized tomography (CT) revealed rim-enhancing hepatic lesions in the which, on biopsy, were consistent with carcinoid tumor and the patient was referred to the nuclear medicine department for further evaluation. What radiopharmaceutical was used to acquire displayed nuclear medicine images?
    (A) Tc-99m tagged red blood cells
    (B) In-111 Octreoscan
    (C) F-18 fluorodeoxyglucose
    (D) Ga-67 citrate

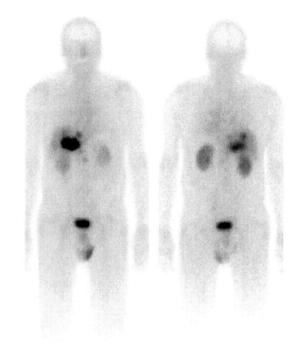

RT   ANT   LT   LT   POST   RT

Fig. 4.14 Nuclear medicine scintigraphy

136. The effects of radiation are usually classified into two categories referred to as stochastic effects and deterministic effects. Which of the following statements describing stochastic and/or deterministic effects is correct?
    (A) Deterministic effect typically has no threshold
    (B) Hemopoietic syndrome is an example of stochastic effects
    (C) Lung cancer is an example of deterministic effects
    (D) The both effects are influenced by the radiation dose

137. The density of ionization reaches a maximum near the end of a particle track and is known as:
(A) Bragg ionization peak
(B) Ionization constant
(C) Stopping power
(D) Bremsstrahlung radiation

138. How far can X-rays and gamma rays travel in the space assuming they will not strike any attenuation objects or medium?
(A) Infinitely
(B) 10 Astronomical units
(C) 1 Astronomical unit
(D) 100 miles

139. A PET scan for myocardial infarction is scheduled to start at 7:00 a.m. Tuesday. The ordered dose of Rubidium-82 is calibrated to contain 350 mCi at 7:00 a.m. The patient is late 5 min for the study and technologist has to calculate how much activity will be available at 7:05 a.m.:
(A) 346.6 mCi
(B) 142.8 mCi
(C) 71.5 mCi
(D) 21.8 mCi

140. The quantitative measurements – left ventricle ejection fraction (LVEF), left ventricle (LV) end-systolic, and end-diastolic volume are possible with gated single photon emission computed tomography myocardial perfusion imaging (gSPECT MPI). Other quantitative measurements, e.g., peak filling rate (PFR) and time to the PFR provide information on:
(A) Left ventricle diastolic function
(B) Left ventricle systolic function
(C) Wall motion
(D) Apical thinning

141. Thyrogen® – thyrotropin alfa for injection – contains a highly purified recombinant form of human:
(A) Thyroid-stimulating hormone (TSH)
(B) Triiodothyronine
(C) Thyroxine
(D) Adrenocorticotropic hormone (ACTH)

142. Pulmonary embolism (PE) is diagnosed when there is more than one subsegment showing:
    (A) Ventilation–perfusion match
    (B) Ventilation–perfusion mismatch
    (C) Poor ventilation
    (D) Poor perfusion

143. The basic signal in positron emission tomography (PET) results from the mutual annihilation of the positron and an electron. An annihilation event leads to the production of:
    (A) Two annihilation protons
    (B) Two annihilation photons and neutrino
    (C) Two annihilation electrons and neutrino
    (D) Two annihilation photons

144. Relatively less activity present at the periphery of the thyroid lobes, where the lobes are thinner due to its pyramidal silhouette, is a normal variation of thyroid images. Asymmetry in thyroid lobe size with the one lobe larger than the other is:
    (A) Is a normal variation
    (B) Is an artifact
    (C) Indicates thyroid pathology
    (D) Requires additional testing

145. Images presented in Fig. 4.15 were obtained from a 52 year old man with chest pain and elevated D-dimer, who was referred to nuclear medicine for a V/Q scan. Findings from the lung ventilation study with Xe-133 are most consistent with:
    (A) Chronic obstructive pulmonary disease (COPD)
    (B) Ribs attenuation
    (C) Lobectomy
    (D) Pulmonary embolism

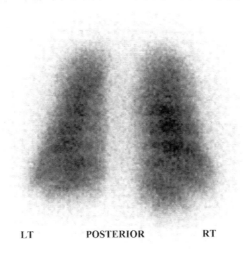

LT   POSTERIOR   RT

Fig. 4.15 Lung ventilation study with Xe-133

146. The nuclear medicine department in clinics and hospitals produces radioactive waste, which is classified as:
    (A) Transuranic (TRU) waste
    (B) Low-level waste (LLW)
    (C) High-level waste (HLW)
    (D) Spent reactor fuel (SRF)

147. In which of the clinical settings does the clearance of Tc-99m methylene diphosphonate (MDP) in the affected extracellular space lag behind that of the remainder of the body?
    (A) Acute osteomyelitis
    (B) Paget's disease
    (C) Lymphatic obstruction
    (D) Ureteral obstruction

148. Molybdenum-99 and Technetium-99 are:
    (A) Isotones
    (B) Isobars
    (C) Isomers
    (D) Isotopes

149. A vial of Tc-99m methylene diphosphonate (MDP) contains 198 mCi in 5.2 ml at 12:00 p.m. Saturday. What was the specific concentration at 11:00 a.m., on the same day? (Precalibration factor is 1.1)

    (A) 217.9 mCi/ml
    (B) 176.4 mCi/ml
    (C) 41.9 mCi/ml
    (D) 33.9 mCi/ml

150. Excess dietary iodine intake, recent iodine contrast, medications containing iodine such as amiodarone can mimic on a thyroid scan:

    (A) Grave's disease
    (B) Multinodular goiter
    (C) Hashimoto's disease
    (D) Autonomously functioning nodule

151. The healthy heart under normal conditions derives more than two-thirds of its energy from:

    (A) Anaerobic glucose metabolism
    (B) Aerobic glucose metabolism
    (C) Oxidative long-chain fatty acids metabolism
    (D) Nonoxidative long-chain fatty acids metabolism

152. A whole-body positron emission tomography/computed tomography (PET/CT) protocol that includes respiratory gated, four dimensional (RG 4D PET/CT) is likely to be recommended for future oncological studies and radiation therapy applications. What are the two essentials guidelines in selection of an appropriate patient for RG 4D PET/CT imaging?

    (A) A regular breathing pattern and good patient collaboration
    (B) A regular breathing pattern and uncompromised renal function
    (C) Good patient collaboration and a regular heart rate
    (D) Good patient collaboration and uncompromised renal function

153. How many atoms decaying per one second are measured by 1 becquerel?

    (A) 1
    (B) 3.7
    (C) 100
    (D) 3.7×100

154. Thyroglossal duct cyst visualization exemplifies the pattern of "extrathyroidal" activity on thyroid scans and in this circumstance I-123 is the preferred agent over Tc-99m because I-123 imaging:

(A) Demonstrates less salivary activity
(B) Is less tissue specific
(C) Allows use of marker
(D) Is less expensive

155. Figure 4.16. A 59 year old man with typical chest pain and dyspnea on exertion with myocardial perfusion treadmill stress test (MPI) – bull's-eye display: label (a) and coronary angiography (PTCA) – coronary tree display – label (b). Which of the following statements correctly describes findings identified with MPI and PTCA?

(A) Normal MPI and normal PTCA
(B) Abnormal MPI in LAD territory and 90% stenosis of circumflex artery on angiogram
(C) Abnormal MPI in CIRC territory and 90% stenosis of circumflex artery on angiogram
(D) Abnormal MPI in RCA territory and 90% stenosis of circumflex artery on angiogram

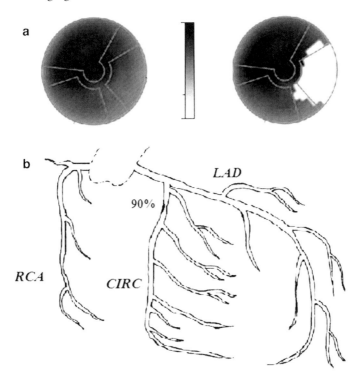

Fig. 4.16 MPI and PTCA (*Illustration by Sabina Moniuszko*)

156. The Medical Internal Radiation Dose (MIRD) committee of the Society of Nuclear Medicine (SNM) designed methods for calculating:
    (A) Threshold doses for deterministic effects
    (B) Therapeutic doses for thyroid ablation
    (C) Internal doses from therapeutic and diagnostic doses
    (D) Diagnostic doses for pediatric patients

157. Chemiadsorption is the mechanism of localization of which of the following radiopharmaceutical?
    (A) Tc-99m macroaggregated albumin (MAA)
    (B) Tc-99m sulfur colloid (SC)
    (C) Tc-99m methylene diphosphonate (MDP)
    (D) Tc-99m mercaptylacetyltriglycine (MAG3)

158. Which of the following devices is used in a gamma-camera to detect radiation?
    (A) Ionization chamber
    (B) Thermoluminescent dosimeter
    (C) Light sensitive film
    (D) Scintillation detector

159. A Tc-99m macroaggregated albumin (MAA) kit is being prepared at 9:00 a.m. to perform ventilation–perfusion (V/Q) scans scheduled for today. If 4 mCi doses are needed at 10:00 a.m., 12:00 p.m., and at 1:00 p.m., what minimum activity should be available at 9:00 a.m. to accommodate the scheduled V/Q scans?
    (A) 23.7 mCi
    (B) 16.5 mCi
    (C) 14.1 mCi
    (D) 12.5 mCi

160. With Zevalin and Bexxar therapies, an unlabeled antibody is infused before the radiolabeled component is administered. What is the purpose of the infusion of unlabeled antibody?
    (A) To saturate CD-20 epitope of nonmalignant B-cells in the circulation and in the spleen
    (B) To confirm normal biodistribution of the labeled antibody
    (C) To determine the therapeutic dose of Zevalin
    (D) To provide a shorter period for tumor perfusion and antibody–epitope binding

161. Amiodarone effect on thyroid function is due to its high iodine contents and because amiodarone is structurally similar to:
    (A) Thyroid-stimulating hormone (TSH)
    (B) Thyroxine
    (C) Methimazole
    (D) Tyrosine

162. Localizing metastatic disease in thyroid cancer patients with F-18 fluorode-oxyglucose (FDG) PET imaging is the primary clinical indication if:
    (A) I-131 whole body scan is negative and thyroglobulin (Tg) is negative
    (B) I-131 whole body scan is negative and thyroglobulin (Tg) is positive
    (C) I-131 whole body scan is positive and thyroglobulin (Tg) is negative
    (D) I-131 whole body scan is positive and thyroglobulin (Tg) is positive

163. The mathematical formula of Butterworth filters contains not only a cutoff frequency number, but also another parameter called the order. The order of the filter adjusts:
    (A) The downslope of the upper part of the filter
    (B) The upperslope of the lower part of the filter
    (C) The upperslope of the upper part of the filter
    (D) The downslope of the lower part of the filter

164. Traditionally solitary pulmonary nodules are defined as focal, round, or oval areas of increased opacity in the lung that measure:
    (A) Less than 1 cm in diameter
    (B) 1–3 cm in diameter
    (C) More than 30 mm in diameter
    (D) 30–50 mm in diameter

165. Figure 4.17. A 49 years old woman with severe upper abdominal pain, vomiting bile, and frequent heartburn was referred to the nuclear medicine department for hepatobiliary scintigraphy. Findings presented in nuclear medicine images are most consistent with the clinical diagnoses of:
    (A) Acute cholecystitis
    (B) Bile leak
    (C) Bile reflux
    (D) Cholelithiasis

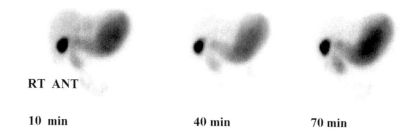

RT ANT

10 min   40 min   70 min

Fig. 4.17 Hepatobiliary scintigraphy

166. All of the following organizations are entitled to develop rules governing transport of radioactive materials EXCEPT:
(A) Department of Transportation (DOT)
(B) Department of Energy (DOE)
(C) FedEx
(D) Postal Service

167. Bremsstrahlung is electromagnetic radiation produced by the acceleration of a charged particle, when deflected by another charged particle. Bremsstrahlung is a word of German origin derived from:
(A) The last name of physicist who discovered the phenomenon
(B) The last name of author who described the phenomenon
(C) Bremsen meaning "to brake" and strahlung meaning "radiation"
(D) Bremsen meaning "to produce" and Strahlung meaning "one lung"

168. A thermoluminescent dosimeter (TLD) and a film badge are the most commonly used personnel radiation exposure monitoring devices. What is the major drawback of their use?
(A) They are fragile
(B) They are environmental unfriendly
(C) They give no immediate readings
(D) They are not reliable

169. Generator elute contains 680 mCi of Tc-99m and 80 μCi Mo-99. How long could this concentration be used before exceeding limit of 0.15 μCi Mo-99/mCi of Tc-99m?
(A) 3.0 h
(B) 169 min
(C) 2.3 h
(D) 68 min

170. There are three stages of disease development in pagetic bone – lytic, intermediate, and sclerotic. In which stage of Paget's disease the bone scintigraphy might NOT show increased radionuclide uptake?
   (A) Intermediate
   (B) In all phases
   (C) Sclerotic
   (D) Lytic

171. Which of the following parenteral routes of medication administrations warrants the fastest absorption of medication from the injection site?
   (A) Subcutaneous injection
   (B) Intramuscular injection
   (C) Intradermal injection
   (D) Intravenous injection

172. Which of the following radionuclides promises to be widely used in positron emission tomography (PET) and will enable innovations in radiopharmaceutical development and advances in the treatment of cancer, in drug development, and in imaging infection?
   (A) Tc-99m
   (B) Tl-201
   (C) Ga-68
   (D) I-131

173. An empty glove box is a commonly used simple way to reduce radiation exposure. A glove box if properly used:
   (A) Contains spills and leaks during vial with radiopharmaceutical opening
   (B) Shields the radioactive dose
   (C) Increases distance between the technologist and the dose
   (D) Reduces time of kit preparation

174. Which of the following two tracers are the most widely used in for the quantification of regional myocardial blood flow with PET?
   (A) F-18-labeled fluorodopamine and C-11-labeled hydroxyephedrine
   (B) F-18 N-methylspiperone and C-11-labeled methiodide salt of quinuclidinyl benzylate
   (C) F-18-labeled glucose and O-15 carbon monoxide
   (D) Oxygen-15-labeled water and nitrogen-13-labeled ammonia

175. Curves of cortical kidney activity are displayed in Fig. 4.18. Graph (a) presents a normal pattern with a prompt increase in activity and spontaneous washout. Curve of cortical kidney activity displayed on graph (b) is described as:

    (A) Dilated nonobstructed pattern
    (B) Blunted response pattern
    (C) Obstructed pattern
    (D) Golden pattern

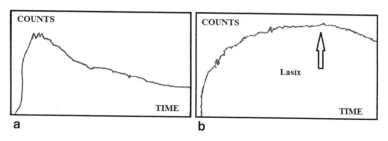

Fig. 4.18 Curves of cortical kidney activity (*Illustration by Sabina Moniuszko*)

176. According to the Department of Transportation/Nuclear Regulatory Commission (DOT/NRC) – Radioactive Materials Shipments Compliance with 49CFR and 10CFR 71, the contents section of the shipping documents must include all of the radionuclides in the container and the activity of the package must be listed in the units of:

    (A) Curies (Ci)
    (B) Becquerels (Bq)
    (C) Disintegrations/s
    (D) Disintegrations/min

177. Visualization of 99mTc-methylene diphosphonate (MDP) bound plasma proteins resulting in images of bowel activity on bone scans can be observed in patients with:

    (A) Proteinuria
    (B) Protein-losing enteropathy
    (C) Irritable bowel syndrome
    (D) Colon cancer

178. A law stating that the radiosensitivity of a tissue depends on the number of undifferentiated cells in the tissue, their mitotic activity, and the length of time they are actively proliferating, is known as:

    (A) The Becquerel rule
    (B) The Curie principle
    (C) The Bergonie–Tribondeau law
    (D) The Roentgen rule

179. Thin layer chromatography (TLC) results were measured in the dose calibrator for a Tc-99m mebrofenin kit. If 3 mCi of free Tc-99m and 55 mCi of Tc-99m mebrofenin were measured in the dose calibrator, what is the percentage of radiopharmaceutical purity?

    (A) 95%
    (B) 93%
    (C) 91%
    (D) 89%

180. The principal functional unit of the kidney is called:

    (A) Pyramid
    (B) Calyx
    (C) Nephron
    (D) Tubule

181. Hyperthyroidism caused by the intentional or accidental ingestion of excess amounts of thyroid hormone called:

    (A) Thyrotoxicosis factitia
    (B) Plummer's disease
    (C) Silent hyperthyroidism
    (D) Subacute thyroiditis

182. F-18-labeled fluorometaraminol, F-18-labeled fluorodopamine, and C-11-labeled hydroxyephedrine are myocardial PET tracers used for imaging:

    (A) Fatty acid metabolism
    (B) Myocardial blood flow
    (C) Presynaptic sympathetic innervations
    (D) Myocardial viability

183. When performing the cardiac shunt study after an IV bolus injection of a radiopharmaceutical, a spiky activity is seen in the lungs followed by a ditch and smaller recirculation peak; unexpected activity appearing before the recirculation peak indicates the presence of:

    (A) Right-to-left shunt
    (B) Left-to-right shunt
    (C) Left-to-left shunt
    (D) Right-to-right shunt

184. Myocardial ischemia could be distinguished from myocardial infarction by analysis of PET images of the perfusion tracer N-13-labeled ammonia and the glucose analogue FDG. Region with "flow-metabolism mismatch" – decreased flow with normal increased FDG activity – represents:

   (A) Viable myocardium
   (B) Hibernating myocardium
   (C) Infarcted myocardium
   (D) Stunned myocardium

185. Figure 4.19.a, b. A 52 year old man with a secondary anemia and LUQ pain referred to nuclear medicine department for gastrointestinal bleeding scintigraphy. Displayed images are obtained after injection of 19.7 mCi of in vitro tagged Tc-99m red blood cells. Findings of the scan are most consistent with:

   (A) No active bleeding
   (B) Active bleeding – transverse colon
   (C) Active bleeding – spleen
   (D) Active bleeding – descending colon

a

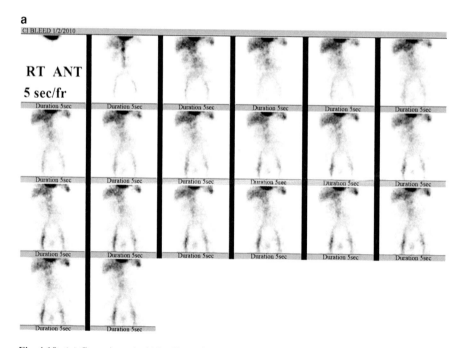

Fig. 4.19 (a) Gastrointestinal bleeding scintigraphy-flow images

b

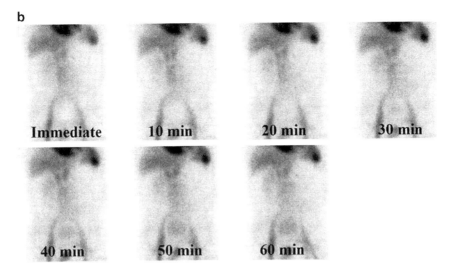

Fig. 4.19 (**b**) Gastrointestinal bleeding scintigraphy-static images

186. The effects of radiation usually associated with exposures to higher levels of radiation and usually incurred over fractions of a second to tens of days are known as:
    (A) Stochastic effects
    (B) Acute effects
    (C) Deterministic effects
    (D) Side effects

187. Gamma rays and X-rays make up part of the electromagnetic spectrum. When travel they can strike an object and all of the following reactions can happen EXCEPT:
    (A) Transmission
    (B) Absorption
    (C) Scattering
    (D) Diversion

188. Filtering in tomographic reconstruction occurs in the frequency domain by reducing high-frequency information (noise). Filters applied in this process are:
    (A) Geometrical figures
    (B) Mathematical formulas
    (C) Mechanical devices
    (D) Standard deviations

189. Gastric emptying study was performed with Tc-99m sulfur colloid mixed with scrambled egg. Counts were derived from region of interest (ROI) drawn over the images obtained immediately and 1 h post consumption of radioactive meal and are listed below:

    - Immediate image: 85,890 cts from anterior view and 81,312 cts from posterior view
    - One hour postconsumption image: 63,250 cts from anterior view and 60,530 cts from posterior view

    What is the fraction of the meal remaining in the stomach at 60 min? (Decay factor is 0.891)

    (A) 83%
    (B) 74%
    (C) 55%
    (D) 17%

190. PET imaging with a substance called Pittsburgh compound B (PIB) which passes through the bloodstream, enters the brain, and attaches itself to beta-amyloid is used in diagnostic workup of patients with:

    (A) Alzheimer's disease
    (B) Parkinson's disease
    (C) Dementia
    (D) Movement disorders

191. Subacute thyroiditis is characterized by an abrupt onset of thyrotoxic symptoms caused by hormone leaks from an inflamed gland. A diagnostic workup will reveal:

    (A) Low serum TSH level, high radionuclide uptake
    (B) High serum TSH level, low radionuclide uptake
    (C) Low serum TSH level, low radionuclide uptake
    (D) High serum TSH level, high radionuclide uptake

192. Brain stimulations, such as motor stimulations, result in hypermetabolism in the area of the brain that is impacted by that stimulation and on PET FDG images this area will light up. If the patient exercises his or her left arm 30 min before the procedure which area of the brain will show increased radiotracer uptake during the PET FDG scan?

    (A) Left motor cortex
    (B) Right motor cortex
    (C) Occipital lobe
    (D) Auditory area

193. A computer language designed for performing complex calculations and dealing with large amount of numeric data called:
  (A) Beginner's All-purpose Symbolic Instruction Code (BASIC)
  (B) COmmon Business-Oriented Language (COBOL)
  (C) Formula Translation (FORTRAN)
  (D) Pascal

194. The reimbursement for cardiac imaging available from The Centers for Medicare & Medicaid Services at the present time is limited to:
  (A) F-18 FDG for myocardial viability, Rb-82 and N-13 ammonia for myocardial perfusion
  (B) F-18 FDG for myocardial viability, C-11 acetate for myocardial oxidative metabolism
  (C) Rb-82 and N-13 ammonia for myocardial perfusion, O-15 water for myocardial blood flow
  (D) O-15 water for myocardial blood flow, C-11 palmitate for myocardial oxidative metabolism

195. Figure 4.20 a, b. A 60 year old man with fever, shortness of breath, and atypical chest pain referred for nuclear medicine ventilation–perfusion scan. Ventilation images were acquired with 12.1 mCi of inhaled Xe-133 and perfusion images with 4.1 mCi of Tc-99m macroaggregated albumin (MAA). Findings of performed lung scintigraphy are most consistent with:
  (A) Normal scan
  (B) Matched left lung defect
  (C) Matched right lung defect
  (D) Unmatched left lung defect

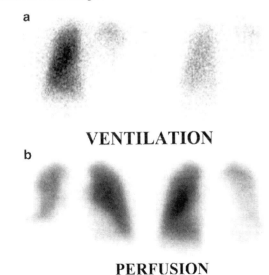

Fig. 4.20 (a) & (b) Nuclear medicine ventilation-perfusion scan

196. According to the NRC/DOT regulations there are three basic types of packages that can be used for radioactive material transport. Which of the following is NOT the type of container listed in the regulations?
    (A) Strong tight container
    (B) Type A containers
    (C) Type B containers
    (D) Type D containers

197. The main treatment options for patients diagnosed with persistent hyperthyroidism are all of the following EXCEPT:
    (A) Antithyroid medications
    (B) Radioactive iodine
    (C) Surgery
    (D) Beta blockers

198. The process of convolution in the spatial domain is equivalent to what process in the frequency space:
    (A) Multiplication
    (B) Subtraction
    (C) Summation
    (D) Division

199. Lung quantitation study was performed on 65-year-old male diagnosed with lung cancer. Counts derived from gamma-camera images are given below. What is the percentage perfusion of the lower lobe of right lung?

    | Right upper lobe | 18,950 counts | Left upper lobe | 13,215 counts |
    | Right middle lobe | 25,345 counts | Left middle lobe | 24,789 counts |
    | Right lower lobe | 47,896 counts | Left lower lobe | 32,720 counts |

    (A) 29%
    (B) 25%
    (C) 15%
    (D) 12%

200. Which of the following statements describing radioisotopes Sr-89, Sm-153, and P-32 in the treatment of bone metastases is FALSE?
    (A) P-32 has rarely been used because marrow toxicity
    (B) Sm-153 has the longest half-life
    (C) The onset of pain relief with Sr-89 occurs 7–20 days after injection
    (D) The onset of pain relief with Sm-153 is quite rapid

201. A small vascular malformation of the gastrointestinal system which is a com-
     mon cause of otherwise unexplained bleeding and anemia is called:

     (A) Angioedema
     (B) Vasculitis
     (C) Angiodysplasia
     (D) Varicosities gut

202. Short axis tomograms of rest and stress myocardial perfusion imaging studies
     are displayed from:

     (A) Apex-to-inferior wall
     (B) Apex-to-base
     (C) Base-to-apex
     (D) Base-to-anterior wall

203. F-18 FDG uptake in tumors correlates with tumor:

     (A) Growth and viability
     (B) Volume and stability
     (C) Size and contractility
     (D) Shape and reproducibility

204. High glucose levels may interfere with tumor targeting due to competitive
     inhibition of FDG uptake by d-glucose. FDG-PET study should not be recom-
     mended when the glucose level in the blood exceeds:

     (A) 120 mg/dl
     (B) 155 mg/dl
     (C) 175 mg/dl
     (D) 200 mg/dl

205. A 71-year-old man with anemia secondary to acute blood loss and recent
     cholecystectomy. Images presented in Fig. 4.21 were acquired after 20.8 mCi
     of Technetium-99m-labeled autologous red cells administration. Images dem-
     onstrate progressive radionuclide accumulation and are most consistent with
     the presence of:

     (A) Active bleeding in the transverse colon
     (B) Abdominal wall hematoma
     (C) Ruptured hemangioma
     (D) Active sigmoidal bleeding

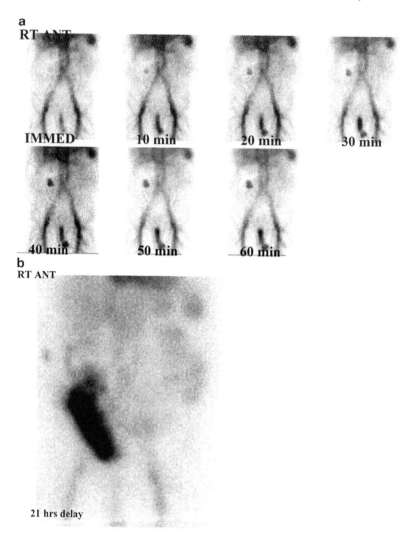

Fig. 4.21 (a) & (b) Gastrointestinal bleeding scintigraphy

206. Acute radiation syndrome (ARS) is defined as an acute illness caused by a dose greater than 50 rads of penetrating radiation to most or all of the body in a short time, usually a matter of minutes. What are the earliest symptoms of ARS?

   (A) Hair loss, alopecia
   (B) Bleeding, bruising
   (C) Nausea, vomiting
   (D) Swelling, necrosis

207. Initial Tl-201 uptake depends on regional myocardial blood flow and extraction fraction though myocardial concentration of Tl-201 changes over time. Described process is known as:

(A) Redistribution
(B) Roll-off phenomenon
(C) Steal phenomenon
(D) Saturation

208. When performing parathyroid scintigraphy and applying dual isotope – thallium/pertechnetate – digital subtraction technique:

(A) Tc-99m thyroid image is subtracted from Tl-201 parathyroid image
(B) Tl-201 thyroid image is subtracted from Tc-99m parathyroid image
(C) Tc-99m parathyroid image is subtracted from Tl-201 thyroid image
(D) Tl-201 parathyroid image is subtracted from Tl-201 thyroid image

209. Tc-99m bulk vial contains 250 mCi at 7:00 a.m. If three 20 mCi doses are withdrawn at 9:00 a.m., 11:00 a.m., and 3:00 p.m., what is the remaining activity in the vial at 3:00 p.m. after the last dose withdraw?

(A) 56 mCi
(B) 140 mCi
(C) 157 mCi
(D) 225 mCi

210. Which of the following injections sites provides the most direct access to route to the superior vena cava (SVC)?

(A) The right median basilic vein
(B) The left median basilic vein
(C) The right cephalic vein
(D) The left cephalic vein

211. The heart is capable of remodeling in response to environmental burden, and a variety of stimuli can induce it to grow or shrink. Which of the following conditions can be responsible for developing cardiac atrophy?

(A) Hypertension
(B) Pregnancy
(C) Bed rest
(D) Stress

212. Most patients with well-differentiated thyroid cancer have a normal life expectancy; however, they have to be closely monitored for local recurrence and distance metastases. Which of the following diagnostic methods are most commonly used for these purposes?
    (A) Computed tomography and ultrasound
    (B) Magnetic resonance imaging and positron emission tomography
    (C) Whole-body radioiodine scanning and serum thyroglobulin level
    (D) Whole-body bone scintigraphy and thyroid radioiodine uptake

213. Bilinear scaling method employed in combined PET/CT scanners software is used to:
    (A) Convert CT image values to PET attenuation coefficients
    (B) Correct image misregistration
    (C) Improve counting statistics of the PET acquisition
    (D) Adjust positional mismatches

214. Radiopharmaceuticals used in imaging of infection and inflammation accumulate in the region of interest because of the locally changed physiologic conditions. An infectious/inflammatory process is characterized by all of the following EXCEPT:
    (A) Influx of white blood cells
    (B) Increased vascular permeability
    (C) Increased blood flow
    (D) Influx of red blood cells

215. The parameter that is a measure of the concentration of tracer within volume of interest in relation to the concentration of tracer in the rest of the body is known as:
    (A) Specific activity
    (B) Standardized uptake value
    (C) Activity curve
    (D) Volume distribution

216. Brain natriuretic peptide (BNP) is secreted by the ventricles of the heart and is commonly elevated in patients diagnosed with congestive heart failure. The effect of BNP is:
    (A) A decrease in blood volume
    (B) An increase in cardiac output
    (C) An increase in BP
    (D) A decrease in RBC count

217. Tc-99m pertechnetate quick allocation in the extracellular fluid is similar to:
    (A) Magnesium
    (B) Calcium
    (C) Iodide
    (D) Sodium

218. An interventional radiology technique in which a light sensitive drug produces a cytotoxic cellular effect within the plaque and "melts" atherosclerotic plaque is called:
    (A) Photoangioplasty
    (B) Phototherapy
    (C) Angiogenesis
    (D) Angioseal

219. Displayed below data were obtained 24 h after ingestion of the 300 µCi I-123 capsules during RAIU study. What is the calculated thyroid uptake?

    300 µCi I-123 capsules –345,890 cpm Background cts –111 cpm
    Thyroid cts   –80,123 cpm   Thigh cts   –5,324 cpm

    24 h decay factor – 0.284

    (A) 22%
    (B) 34%
    (C) 45%
    (D) 76%

220. Acute coronary syndrome (ACS) is the consequence of disruption of a vulnerable coronary artery plaque and includes all of the following clinical presentations EXCEPT:
    (A) ST segment elevation myocardial infarction
    (B) Non-ST segment elevation MI
    (C) Unstable angina
    (D) Chronic CAD

Answers

1. A – White cells in the urine

   Hematuria – blood in the urine, proteinuria – protein in the urine, cylindruria – microscopic casts in the urine.
   (Early and Sodee 1995)

2. C – Assist in diagnosing arrhythmias

   The quantitative measurements possible with gated SPECT MPI include the following: perfusion – extent and severity of defect, segmental and summed scores; function global and regional – LVEF, EDV, ESV, peak filling rate, and time PFR; other – TID ratio, LV mass, LV eccentricity.
   (Zaret and Beller 2005)

3. Convert CT image values to PET attenuation coefficients

   The attenuation correction factor depends on the energy of the photons; derived from ~70 keV CT X-ray photons must be scaled to the 511 keV PET photons.
   (Saha 2005)

4. A – To inhibit secretion of pertechnetate into the bowel

   Potassium perchlorate – inhibits localization of pertechnetate in ectopic mucosa-should be administered after the radionuclide study to reduce radiation dose to the thyroid.
   (Chistian et al. 2004)

5. A – The left bundle branch

   In the left bundle branch block ventricular contraction is not completely synchronized due to a block in conduction of an electrical impulse to the ventricles and resulting in early activation of the right side of the septum and the right ventricular myocardium before left ventricle activation. Asynchrony in ventricles contraction can result in a septal defect on perfusion imaging which may be mistaken for myocardial infarction or ischemia.
   (Zaret and Beller 2005)

6. A – The radiation must be penetrating

   High-energy X-rays, gamma rays, and neutrons are penetrating radiation.
   (CDC 2010)

7. A – 0.6–4 mm

   In a PET camera of diameter 1 m and active transaxial FOV of 0.6 m the range of positron results in a positional inaccuracy of 2–3 mm.
   (Alessi et al. 2010)

8. C – The anterior surface is up and the right side is on the left
   (English and Brown 1990)

9. D – 14
   (Appendix A, Formula 12)

10. C – Sarcomas
    A sarcoma is a cancer that arises from transformed connective tissue cells.
    (Christian 2004)

11. A – Greater than 1.0
    (Early and Sodee 1995)

12. C – Antihypertensives
    Antihypertensive drugs that deplete norepinephrine stores or inhibit reuptake, e.g., reserpine, should be discontinued for five biological half-lives prior to AdreView administration.
    (GE Healthcare 2010)

13. D – 5–7 o'clock
    The region from 7 to 1 o'clock is supplied by the LAD, from 1 to 5 o'clock by LCX; however, there is a good deal of individual variability.
    (English and Brown 1990)

14. D – Perfusion, parenchymal uptake, gallbladder ejection fraction
    (Ziessman 2009)

15. C – Cystic duct obstruction
    Acute cholecystitis is the most common clinical indication for hepatobiliary scintigraphy and the usual cause of acute cholecystitis is obstruction of the cystic duct.
    (Ziessman 2009)

16. C – Radon is the most frequent cause of lung cancer
    The most common cause of lung cancer is tobacco smoke. According to the U.S. Environmental Protection Agency, estimated 12% of lung-cancer deaths is attributable to radon gas, or about 20,000 lung cancer-related deaths annually in the USA, what makes radon the second leading cause of lung cancer in the USA.
    (Wikipedia 2010)

17. C – Delta ray

The charged particle giving rise to delta rays generally is relatively large, such as an alpha particle but may also be a high-speed electron.
(NCRP 2010)

18. C – Brain

The brain is considered a rigid organ since the shape and size of the brain stay fixed because of the bony skull surrounding it.
(Saha 2005)

19. D – 8,393 dpm

(Appendix A, Formula 15)

20. C – Hepatobiliary

During the first 24 h 10–25% of radionuclide is excreted by the kidneys.
(Bleeker-Rovers et al. 2009)

21. B – Hypertension

Remaining identified factors were: dietary risk, lack of physical activity, diabetes, cardiac causes, stress, and depression.
(Interstroke 2010)

22. A – Gamma probe and/or blue dye

The surgeon identifies and removes the LNs and the pathologist determines whether the metastases are present.
(Pitman 2005)

23. B – Larger with a lower activity concentration

PVE affecting tumor size is especially challenging when PET is used to assist in radiotherapy treatment planning. The borders of a lesion as seen on a PET image may cover more than the real metabolically active part of the tumor. CT image usually clearly shows the tumor contours but the CT image does not delineate the metabolically active part of the tumor.
(Soret et al. 2007)

24. A – Hypertrophic pulmonary osteoarthropathy

HPO is most often seen in the femora, tibiae, and wrists and it is often secondary to chronic lung, e.g., bronchogenic carcinoma and heart conditions.
(Gnanasegaran et al. 2009)

25. D – Dyskinetic left ventricle

Dyskinesis – seen there on the anteroapical surfaces – refers to paradoxic bulging of a small portion of the left ventricle wall with systole.
(Zaret and Beller 2005)

26. A – Patient information booklets

Absorbed dose is the energy absorbed per unit mass at a given point. Effective dose is not physical quantity but is calculated by multiplying actual organ doses by each organ's relative radiosensitivity (risk weighting factors) – to developing cancer – and summing up the total of all the numbers.
(Christian 2004)

27. D – A straight line

The slope of the line is the decay constant l (gamma) of the radionuclide.
(Springer 2010)

28. B – LUT

Lookup table section of the image display: the original data in image memory is not affected by the process, so the original image data can be readily retrieved in cases where an unsatisfactory output image is obtained.
(Wikipedia June 19, 2010)

29. C – 56,174 and 57,606 cpm
(Appendix A, Formula 13)

30. C – Sternal foramina

The photopenic area is more prominent on SPECT images and should not be mistaken for an osteolytic lesion.
(Gnanasegaran et al. 2009)

31. B – Clopidogrel

Plavix is in a class of medications called antiplatelet drugs. Because Plavix slows clotting it will take longer than usual to stop bleeding. Warfarin (Coumadin) and commonly used aspirin also affect bleeding time.
(Perry and Potter 2006)

32. Anterior

Anterior view with the head straight allows for comparison of right and left carotid flow.
(Zuckier and Kolano 2008)

33. A – Suppresses low counts

An exponential relationship provides background subtraction.
(Christian et al. 2004)

34. D – 1 ml/min

Nuclear medicine imaging techniques allow detecting active bleeding at a rate
of greater than 0.3 ml/min.
(Howarth 2006)

35. D – RPO

Lead markers of known length are used to identify the right inferior costal
margin and midclavicular line. Markers can also be used to calibrate the pixel
size for organ size measurement.
(Early and Sodee 1995)

36. B – 2–20 Gy/h
(Early and Sodee 1995)

37. A – I-123 is reactor and I-131 is cyclotron produced

I-131 is produced from nuclear reactor neutron irradiation of a natural tellu-
rium target. I-123 is produced in a cyclotron by proton irradiation of enriched
xenon.
(Early and Sodee 1995)

38. D – Attenuation correction

The blank scan is not a correction; rather it is used with the transmission data
in the calculation of attenuation correction factors. The blank scan is obtained
daily using transmission rod sources and as such is a good source of quality
control data.
(Saha 2005)

39. D – 5 HVLs and 0.5 cm

Divide 25 by two times 5 to achieve desired exposure rate and multiply 5
(HVLs) by 0.10 mm. (HVL of Ga-67)
(Appendix A, Formula 17)

40. D – Antegrade and retrograde

Blood movement in either direction makes difficult identification of the apparent site of bleeding.
(Howarth 2006)

41. C – Accretion
    (Sircar 2008)

42. D – Small bowel transit time is slower
    Small bowel has also a greater tendency for both antegrade and retrograde extravasated blood movement with peristalsis making detection and localization of bleeding in small bowel even more difficult.
    (Howarth 2006)

43. A – SUV calculation
    The calibration correction is applied to adapt the reconstructed image pixel values into activity concentration.
    (Saha 2005)

44. A – Optional
    Delay imaging can be performed up to 24 h.
    (Ford et al. 1999)

45. C – Active bleeding – descending colon
    (Early and Sodee 1995)

46. C – 85% of the effective dose to the patient population
    (Mettler et al. 2008)

47. A – Apyrogenicity
    The physicochemical tests are used to determine the chemistry, purity, and the integrity of a formulation, while the biological tests ascertain the sterility and apyrogenicity of the radiopharmaceutical.
    (Vallabhajosula et al. 2010)

48. C – 110 min
    F-18 is a fluorine radioisotope which is an important source of positrons (counterparts of the electrons)
    (Wahl 2009)

49. A – 7 mCi
    Decay initial given activity of 423 mCi at 10:00 A.M. Monday to 10:00 A.M. Tuesday and subtract 80 mCi. Use answer obtained from 10:00 A.M. Tuesday decay/subtraction to get answer for 110 mCi at 10:00 A.M. Thursday. Follow the same process to obtain answer for 130 mCi at 10:00 A.M. Friday.
    (Appendix A, Formula 25)

50. A – Hyperparathyroidism

Hyperparathyroidism is caused by overproduction of parathyroid hormone most commonly by single parathyroid adenoma (primary hyperthyroidism) or because of another disease that affects the glands' function (secondary hyperparathyroidism). Symptoms of hyperthyroidism include depression, loss of appetite, nausea, vomiting, constipation, etc.
(Gnanasegaran et al. 2009)

51. C – Gray matter

Gray matter contains mostly nerve cell bodies and unmyelinated fibers. The white matter of the brain contains nerve fibers.
(Early and Sodee 1995)

52. Mucinous adenocarcinoma

(Gnanasegaran et al. 2009)

53. A – –1,000
(Wahl 2009)

54. D – 4 h after injection
(Love and Palestro 2010)

55. D – A

(Christian et al. 2004)
A MuGA scan may be called by other names, such as Radionuclide Angiography, Gated Blood Pool Scan, multigated acquisition, Cardiac Blood Pool Scan, Ejection Fraction Study, and Radionuclide Ventriculogram.

56. B – 20–40 mSv
(Brix et al. 2005)

57. B – I-124 and I-125

Significant image degradation may be caused by Compton scatter and septal penetration from high-energy photons emitted by I-124.
(Vallabhajosula et al. 2010)

58. C – IR requires higher counts density

The foremost limitation for introducing iterative reconstruction technique in nuclear medicine has been computation time, which is much longer for iterative techniques than for FBP. Iterative algorithms allow integration of important corrections, e.g., attenuation and scatter.
(Wahl 2009)

59. C – 22 h and 3 days
    (Appendix A, Formula 18)

60. C – Gallium-67 citrate
    (Love and Palestro 2010)

61. B – Angioplasty
    PTCA – percutaneous transluminal coronary angioplasty – a procedure with a
    balloon-tipped catheter to enlarge a narrowing in a coronary artery.
    (AHA 2010)

62. B – Gallbladder function
    (Ziessman 2009)

63. B – CZT-based SPECT cameras have Tc-99m energy resolution of 9–10% vs.
    5.7% of Anger's
    (ASNC information statement 2010)

64. C – Lateral views
    (Howarth 2006)

65. C – Patient B has rib fractures, patient A has bone metastases
    The ribs fractures on a bone scintigraphy are seen as focal/perpendicular, sev-
    eral in row areas of increased radiotracer uptake. The ribs metastases are paral-
    lel to the ribs and vary in location.
    (Early and Sodee 1995)

66. D – Different patients
    (U.S. REMM 2010)

67. D – Liquid scintillation counter
    (Saha 2006)

68. B – PACS
    Picture archiving and communication systems. DICOM is the common image
    file format for PACS image transfer and storage. Nonimage data, e.g., such as
    scanned documents, may also be incorporated using, e.g., PDF file format.
    (Christian et al. 2004)

69. C – 170,100 µCi
     (Appendix A, Formula 9B)

70. B – Hepatocellular carcinoma
     The accumulation of FDG in well-differentiated hepatocellular carcinoma
     (HCC) may be similar to that of the surrounding normal liver, making the
     detection of HCCs not easy.
     (Lin and Alavi 2009)

71. A – Gastric mucosa
     The popular rule of 2s describing Meckel's diverticulum: 2% of the population
     – 2 ft from the ileocecal valve – 2 in. long – 2% of patients are symptomatic,
     males are two times as likely to be affected, there are two types of common
     ectopic tissue gastric and pancreatic, and the most common age at clinical pre-
     sentation is age 2.
     (Christian et al. 2004)

72. D – Low mitotic rate
     (Wahl 2009)

73. A – White noise
     White noise or Poison statistical noise has approximately the same amplitude
     at all frequencies and is added to the profiles. "White noise" name by analogy
     to the energy spectrum of white light.
     (Groch and Erwin 2000)

74. A – Shunt glucose to skeletal and cardiac muscles
     Insulin is a natural hormone made by the pancreas that is essential for regulat-
     ing carbohydrate and fat metabolism in the body.
     (Lin and Alavi)

75. A – C
     (Christian et al. 2004)

76. A – With the birth of another child
     (SNM Guideline 2002)

77. C – Rb-82
     Each PET radionuclide produces its positron with a different energy – higher
     energy particles travel greater path lengths before annihilation process.
     (Christian et al. 2004)

78. C – High counts flood

PSF (Point Spread Function) measures the blur of a hot spot and LSF (Line Spread Function) depicts the counts density of capillary tube in a gamma-camera image. (Halama 2010)

79. A – 3.8 mCi/ml

Obtain concentration and decay that concentration to get answer, or decay first and then get concentration.

(Appendix A, Formulas 28A and 25)

80. A – PET/CT has higher resolution and visualized physiologic variability is more prominent

(Lin and Alavi 2009)

81. D – Is longer with an increase in vagal inputs

The vagus nerve innervates the sinoatrial node and acts to lower the heart rate. Vagal (parasympathetic) hyperstimulation predisposes to bradyarrhythmias. (Podrid 2008)

82. C – Varies with the density of the breast

(Zaret and Beller 2005)

83. C – Chang attenuation correction

This method is most useful in the brain and abdomen imaging where the attenuation can be considered uniform.

(Groch and Erwin 2000)

84. A – Is more diffuse than breast attenuation artifact

(Zaret and Beller 2005)

85. B – Septal wall

(Zaret and Beller 2005)

86. A – Radiolytic decomposition of water in a cell

(NRC 2010)

87. B – F-18

(Christian et al. 2004)

88. A – Convert the CT image into an attenuation map

In order for the CT image to be used in the attenuation correction algorithm, the CT numbers must be converted to attenuation coefficients at the energy of the SPECT radionuclide.

(Lin and Alavi 2009)

89. B – 76%

(Appendix A, Formula 38B)

90. A – RV overload

Flattening of the interventricular septum (D-shape left ventricle) in addition to high right ventricle tracer uptake and increased right ventricle volume found on gated SPECT studies strongly correlates with right ventricular overload.
(Zaret and Beller 2005)

91. D – The QRS duration is influenced by heart rate
(Podrid 2008)

92. D – The diaphragm is pushed down
(Zaret and Beller 2005)

93. D – Amplitude of the signal pulses is dependent on the energy of the incoming radiation

The cutie-pie ionization detector has a signal that depends on the energy of the detected X-rays or gamma rays and is for that reason directly related to the exposure for all radionuclides. Cutie-pie is a low-sensitivity ionization detector and is designed for use in high exposure areas.
(Halama 2010)

94. A – Septum

LBBB is a conduction abnormality in which the signal cannot pass through the left bundle branch and as a result conduction to the LV comes from the right ventricle and is delayed. The apparent defect results from compromise of dia-stolic blood flow due to the delayed septal contraction and is augmented by increasing heart rate, e.g., during exercise.
(Zaret and Beller 2005)

95. A – Sphincter of Oddi

Sphincter of Oddi functions as a one-way valve to allow bile and pancreatic secretions to enter the bowel, while preventing the contents of the bowel from backing up into these ducts.
(Christian et al. 2004)

96. C – Dose of about 3 mSv per year

These natural "background" doses vary throughout the country.
(Radiologyinfo.org 2010)

97. A – Alpha-particle emitters
(Kassis 2008)

98. B – 0.002 microcurie/g

This definition does not specify a quantity, only a concentration. Be aware that the above definition of radioactive material applies only for transportation purposes.
(NRC 2010)

99. A – 1.5 ml

(Appendix A, Formulas 28A and 25)

100. C – Partial volume effect

(Zaret and Beller 2005)

101. C – Apoptosis

Pinocytosis is the process by which extracellular fluid is taken into a cell. Endocytosis is the process by which cells absorb molecules.
(Wikipedia 2010)

102. C – 6

(Zaret and Beller 2005)

103. A – The background counting rate

The background exposure should be measured daily in an area out-of-the-way from radioactive sources within the nuclear medicine facility.
(Zanzonico 2008)

104. A – 3%

The blood clearance of Tc-99m MDP is high. Within 1 h, with normal renal function, more than 30% of the unbound complex has undergone glomerular filtration.
(Christian et al. 2004)

105. B – Brain death scintigraphy

Under certain circumstances, confirmatory tests can be used to shorten the clinical observation before a patient can be declared brain dead. Cerebral scintigraphy is a reliable and widely available test recommended by the American Academy of Neurology and the American Academy of Pediatrics.
(Zuckier and Kolano 2005)

106. C – Four times greater

(Medscape Radiology 2010)

107. C – Oxygen-15

(Kassis 2008)

108. C – Co-60

Co-57 with a half-life of 271.79 days is employed for instrumentation QC in nuclear medicine.
Although Co-60 β-decay energy is low and easily shielded Co-60 is not used for QC purposes.
(Zanzonico 2008)

109. C – 159 mCi

(Appendix A, Formula 27)

110. D – The incidence and extent of arrhythmias on electrocardiogram (ECG)

(Zaret and Beller 2005)

111. B – The right atrium from the right ventricle

(Frohlich 2001)

112. A – Ventilation–perfusion scanning and pulmonary angiography

Prospective investigation of pulmonary embolism diagnosis III (PIOPED III) follows PIOPED I and PIOPED and evaluates Gadolinium-enhanced MRA in combination with venous phase magnetic resonance venography for the diagnosis of acute PE.
(ClinicalTrials.gov 2010)

113. C – 37 kBq

Enormously high sensitivity of current scintillation well counters results from the use of a thick crystal and a well-type counting geometry of well counters; at higher activities, because of dead-time counting losses measurements become inaccurate.
(Zanzonico 2008)

114. B – *Dextrocardia*

Mesocardia is an uncommon location of the heart, with the apex in the midline of the thorax.
(TheFreeDictionary 2010)

115. A – Left circumflex artery (LCX)

(Christian et al. 2004)

116. A – To be more restrictive than the Federal guidelines.

(Nuclear Medicine Tutorials 2010)

117. A – Strontium-82
(Wahl 2009)

118. A – V/Q scan
D-dimer is a small protein fragment present in the blood after a blood clot is degraded and its concentration may help diagnose thrombotic disorders. A negative result practically excludes thromboembolic disease.
(Stein et al. 2007)

119. A – 312 mCi
Obtain precalibration of given activity for each different time given in the problem and add all three precalibrated activity answers to obtain accumulative activity needed. Precalibration activity is always more than activity given; therefore, depending on the half-life answer could be estimated.
(Appendix A, Formula 25)

120. C – Tagged WBCs for osteomyelitis diagnosis
In a WBC's scintigraphy white blood cells are separated from the rest of the blood sample and then mixed with a small amount of Tc-99m or Indium-111. About 2 or 3 h later, the tagged white blood cells are reinjected and imaging is performed 2–24 h later.
(Early and Sodee 1995)

121. D – Abdominal aorta
Kidneys, bladder, duodenum, sigmoid colon, and pancreas also lie in the extraperitoneal space.
(Wikipedia 2010)

122. A – ≤2%
Hyperthyroidism is caused by disruption of thyroid follicles and release of excessive amounts of thyroid hormone into the blood. Damaged thyroid cells are unable to concentrate iodine (low or minimal uptake).
(Sarkar 2006)

123. C – Inverse Fourier transform
(Christian et al. 2004)

124. B – Thymus
The T is for thymus – a lymphoid organ situated in the center of the upper chest just behind the sternum.
(Goldsmith 2010)

125. C – Multinodular goiter

A multinodular goiter (MNG) is a thyroid gland that is commonly enlarged and contains multiple thyroid nodules.
(Christian et al. 2004)

126. Deoxyribonucleic acid (DNA)

DNA provides the instructions for building proteins required for the growth, development, and reproduction of an organism.
(Kassis 2008)

127. D – Iodination
(Early and Sodee 1995)

128. D – Fourier transform, filtering, inverse Fourier transform, backprojection

The Fourier transform of the projection data into the frequency space is allowing for more efficient filtering of the data.
(Groch and Erwin 2000)

129. B – 10 mCi

No need to utilize concentration in this problem since its just extra information, simply decay 55 mCi to 1:00 p.m. and subtract 25 mCi to obtain the answer.
(Appendix A, Formula 25)

130. A – Rituximab

Rituximab is a man-made antibody that was developed using cloning and recombinant DNA technology from human and murine (mice or rat) genes.
(Goldsmith 2010)

131. C – The inferior angle of the scapula
(Frohlich 1993)

132. D – Hyperemic flow velocity in diseased artery to that of normal artery

Hyperemic flow velocity to the resting flow velocity distal to the stenosis is called absolute CFR.
(Zaret and Beller 2005)

133. D – In-111-labeled diethylenetriamine pentaacetic acid (DTPA) aerosol

Technegas – an ultrafine Tc-99m-labeled solid graphic particles generated in a furnace at high temperature is the superior imaging agent especially in patients with obstructive lung disease.
(Bajc et al. 2010)

134. D – Phenobarbital

Phenobarbital increases bilirubin conjugation and excretion, enhancing bile flow, and has been used to differentiate between biliary atresia vs. neonatal hepatitis.
(Ziessman 2009)

135. B – In-111 Octreoscan

The administered average dose of In-111 Octreoscan is 6.0 mCi (222 MBq) and whole-body anterior and posterior images are acquired at 4 and 24 h with optional SPECT scan at 24 h after radiopharmaceutical injection.
(Christian et al. 2004)

136. D – The both effects are influenced by the radiation dose
(U.S. Environmental Protection Agency 2010)

137. A – Bragg ionization peak
(Wikipedia 2010)

138. A – Infinitely
(Early and Sodee 1995)

139. D – 21.8 mCi
(Appendix A, Formula 25)

140. A – LV diastolic function

Diastole is referring to the time of relaxation and dilatation of ventricles during which they fill with blood.
(Zaret and Beller 2005)

141. A – Thyroid-stimulating hormone (TSH)

The amino acid sequence of thyrotropin alfa is identical to that of human pituitary thyroid-stimulating hormone.
(Thyrogen 2010)

142. B – Ventilation–perfusion mismatch

Emboli, which are commonly multiple, occlude the arteries causing lobar, segmental, or subsegmental perfusion defects within still ventilated areas.
(Bajc et al. 2010)

143. B – Two annihilation photons and neutrino
(Wahl 2009)

144. A – Is a normal variation

Each thyroid lobes measures approximately 5×2 cm, and the gland generally weighs 15–30 g.
(Smith and Oates 2004)

145. B – Ribs attenuation

Gamma energies of Xe-133: 81 keV (38%), 35 keV (7%), 31 keV (38%).
(Wikipedia 2010)

146. B – Low-level waste (LLW)

LLW-waste generated by all radioisotope production, purification, and applications, e.g., NM practice, biomedical research, production of radiopharmaceuticals by private companies.
(Lombardi 1999)

147. C – Lymphatic obstruction
(Gnanasegaran et al. 2009)

148. B – Isobars
(Saha 2004)

149. C – 41.9 mCi/ml
(Appendix A, Formula 27)

150. C – Hashimoto's disease

In Hashimoto's disease immune system attacks own thyroid gland and resulting inflammation often leads to an underactive thyroid gland (hypothyroidism). Hashimoto's disease is the most common cause of hypothyroidism in the USA.
(Smith and Oates 2004)

151. C – Oxidative long-chain fatty acids metabolism

In ischemic myocardium oxidative metabolism of FA is suppressed and the myocardium switches to anaerobic glucose metabolism.
(Wahl 2009)

152. A – A regular breathing pattern and good patient collaboration

Movement reduces image quality and quantitative accuracy for diagnostic purposes and compromises the ability to define accurate target volumes.
(HeathImaging.com 2010)

153. A – 1

One Bq is defined as the activity of a quantity of radioactive material in which one nucleus decays per second. Bq is a small unit and multiples are commonly used: kBq (kilobecquerel, 10^3 Bq), MBq (megabecquerel, 10^6 Bq), GBq (gigabecquerel, 10^9 Bq), etc.

(Early and Sodee 1995)

154. A – Demonstrates less salivary activity

Substernal goiter, lingual thyroid, a prominent pyramidal lobe are other examples of ectopic thyroid tissue.

155. C – Abnormal MPI in CIRC territory and 90% stenosis of circumflex artery on angiogram

The circumflex coronary artery (CIRC, LCX) is a branch of the left main coronary artery (LMCA). The CIRC moves away from the left anterior descending (LAD) and wraps around to the back of the heart. Figure 4.16 shows that there was excellent correlation between the location of the abnormality on MPI and on the subsequent coronary angiography.

(Zaret and Beller 2005)

156. C – Internal doses from therapeutic and diagnostic doses

MIRD – medical internal radiation dose – method is the most widely used way for calculating internal doses.

(Lombardi 1999)

157. C – Tc-99m methylene diphosphonate (MDP)

99mTc-MDP binds via chemiadsorption to hydroxyapatite crystals within mineral deposits in soft tissues and bones.

(Christian et al. 2004)

158. D – Scintillation detector

A thermoluminescent dosimeter (TLD) measures ionizing radiation exposure by measuring the amount of visible light emitted (luminescence) from a crystal in the detector when the crystal is heated (thermo).

(Early and Sodee 1995)

159. B – 16.5 mCi

Obtain precalibration of given activity for each different time given in the problem and add all three precalibrated activity answers to obtain accumulative activity needed. Precalibration activity is always more than activity given; therefore, depending on the half-life answer could be estimated.

(Appendix A, Formula 25)

160. A – To saturate CD-20 epitope of nonmalignant B-cells in the circulation and in the spleen

    (Goldsmith 2010)

161. B – Thyroxine

    Amiodarone is an antiarrhythmic drug that has been successful in treating many arrhythmias where other antiarrhythmic drugs have failed.
    (Mycek and Harvey 2008)

162. B – I-131 whole body scan is negative and thyroglobulin (Tg) is positive

    Thyroglobulin (Tg) can only be made by the thyroid tissue – the remaining normal part or the tumorous metastatic part. When a patient has had their thyroid completely removed, the measurement of Tg in a blood can be used to check whether there is any residual tumor present.
    (Lin and Alavi 2009)

163. A – The downslope of the upper part of the filter

164. B – 1–3 cm in diameter

    There is limited evidence that PET may be accurate in nodules smaller than 1 cm.
    (Lin and Alavi 2009)

165. C – Bile reflux

    Bile reflux (duodenogastric reflux, biliary reflux) is caused by upward flows of bile from the liver into the stomach and esophagus. Gastroesophageal reflux disease (GERD) happens when the stomach acids flow into the esophagus.
    (Christian et al. 2004)

166. C – FedEx
    (NRC 2010)

167. C – Bremsen meaning "to brake" and Strahlung meaning "radiation"
    (Wikipedia 2010)

168. C – They give no immediate readings
    (Early and Sodee 1995)

169. C – 2.3 h
    (Appendix A, Formula 30C)

170. B – Sclerotic

Mature lesions might not show up on bone scans because pagetic activity has subsided.

(Chaffins 2007)

171. D – Intravenous injection

Dermis and subcutaneous tissue are not as richly supplied with blood vessels as muscles and as a result the rate of medication absorption from these sites is slower.

(Perry and Potter 2006)

172. C – Ga-68

Ga-68 is available from an in house generator making Ga-68 radiopharmacy independent of an onsite cyclotron. Ga-68 has a half-life of 68 min and decays by 89% through positron emission.

(Sathekge 2008)

173. A – Contains spills and leaks during vial with radiopharmaceutical opening

(Early and Sodee 1995)

174. D – Oxygen-15-labeled water and nitrogen-13-labeled ammonia

Oxygen-15-labeled water is freely diffusible tracer; nitrogen-13-labeled ammonia is retained in myocardial tissue.

(Wahl 2009)

175. B – Blunted response pattern

Kidneys show gradually increasing activity and blunted response to Lasix administration caused by, e.g., a partial obstruction, poor renal function, or dehydration. Indeterminate or equivocal renal scintigraphy results will be reported.

(Christian et al. 2004)

176. B – Becquerels (Bq)

Activity must be listed in the units of SI system but traditional units, such as mCi, may be used if they are in parentheses in addition to the Bq units.

177. B – Protein-losing enteropathy

Protein-losing enteropathy (PLE) is a pathophysiologic process manifested by excessive loss of plasma proteins into the gastrointestinal lumen. Substantial protein binding of Tc-99m MDP – varying from around 25–30% immediately after tracer administration and increasing to 45–55% at 4 h and 60–70% at 24 h – explains observed bowel visualization.

(Gnanasegaran et al. 2009)

178. C – The Bergonie–Tribondeau law

The generalization of the Law of Bergonie and Tribondeau is that tissues which are young and rapidly growing are most likely radiosensitive.
(Early and Sodee 1995)

179. A – 95%

(Appendix A, Formula 32A)

180. C – Nephron

There are approximately two million nephrons in the two kidneys. Each nephron is composed of the glomerulus, Bowman's capsule, and a series of tubules that lead from the capsule to the renal pelvis.
(Frohlich 1993)

181. A – Thyrotoxicosis factitia

TSH is suppressed, T 3 and T 4 levels are elevated, I-123 uptake is absent.
(Andreoli et al. 2001)

182. C – Presynaptic sympathetic innervations

C-11 palmitate is used to assess the rate of fatty acids metabolism; oxygen-15-labeled water and nitrogen-13-labeled ammonia are used for the quantification of regional myocardial blood flow.
(Wahl 2009)

183. B – Left-to-right shunt

From a time activity curve of lung activity a quantitative estimation of shunting can be acquired.
(Christian et al. 2004)

184. A – Viable myocardium

During hypoxia and ischemia affected myocardium uses glucose in preference to fatty acids as the energy source.
(Lin and Alavi 2009)

185. C – Active bleeding – spleen

Flow study and static images demonstrate progressive accumulation of activity in the region of the tip of the spleen consistent with a focal bleed.
(Early and Sodee 1995)

186. C – Deterministic effects
     (U.S. Environmental Protection Agency 2010)

187. D – Diversion
     (Early and Sodee 1995)

188. B – Mathematical formulas
     (Christian et al. 2004)

189. A – 83%
     (Appendix A, Formula 35A)

190. A – Alzheimer's disease
     Close relative of the beta-amyloid protein may be a major reason in the amyloid cascade hypothesis in Alzheimer's disease pathology.
     (Wahl 2009)

191. C – Low serum TSH level, low radionuclide uptake
     (Andreoli et al. 2001)

192. B – Right motor cortex
     The occipital lobe is the visual processing center of the human brain.
     (Wahl 2009)

193. C – Formula Translation (FORTRAN)
     BASIC has been one of the most commonly used computer programming languages, an easy step for students to learn before more powerful languages such as FORTRAN.
     (Christian et al. 2004)

194. A – F-16 FDG for myocardial viability, Rb-82 and N-13 ammonia for myocardial perfusion
     Nitrogen N-13 ammonia up to 40 millicuries, Fluorodeoxyglucose F-18 FDG up to 45 millicuries, and Rubidium Rb-82 up to 60 millicuries – all diagnostic, per study dose.
     (Medicare 2010)

195. C – Matched right lung defect

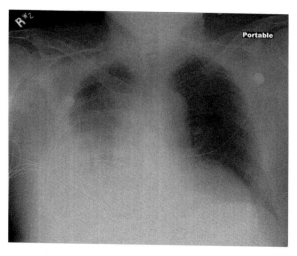

Fig. 4.22 Chest X-ray

Perfusion scan demonstrates in the right mid and lower lung zone matching with ventilation scan and chest X-ray findings (Fig. 4.22 moderate to large right pleural effusion). Results of the pulmonary scintigraphy were reported as "low probability for pulmonary embolism."
(Christian et al. 2004)

196. D – Type D containers

A strong tight container is designed to survive normal transportation handling.
Type A container is designed to survive normal transportation handling and minor accidents; type B container must be able to survive severe accidents.
(NRC 2010)

197. D – Beta blockers

Beta blockers help to control the symptoms of hyperthyroidism.
(Andreoli et al. 2001)

198. A – Multiplication in the frequency domain

This means that any filtering performed by the convolution operation in the spatial domain can be performed by a simple multiplication when Fourier transformed into the frequency domain.
(Christian et al. 2004)

199. A – 29%
   (Appendix A, Formula 37)

200. B – Sm-153 has the longest half-life
   Half-life of Sm-153 is 1.9 days which is much shorter than that of Sr-89 (50.6 days) and P-32 (14.3 days).
   (Saha 2004)

201. C – Angiodysplasia
   Angiodysplasia is a condition in which the blood vessels are dilated, thin and their walls have little or no smooth muscle.
   (Emedicine 2010)

202. A – Apex-to-base
   (Zaret and Beller 2005)

203. A – Growth and viability
   FDG is an analogue of glucose and its uptake depends on an increased glyco-lytic activity in neoplastic cells.
   (Lin and Alavi 2009)

204. D – 200 mg/dl
   Blood glucose level is an important factor affecting the normal liver FDG uptake in nondiabetic patients. In the case of higher glucose level, liver FDG uptake is elevated especially in the delayed image.
   (Lin and Alavi 2009)

205. Abdominal wall hematoma
   CT scan – Fig. 4.23 revealed the presence of inhomogenous soft tissue density and enlargement entire rectus muscle suggesting rectus sheath hematoma (arrow).
   This case provides a fine example for the use of Tc-99m RBC's scintigra-phy in the detection and possible follow-up of active soft tissue bleeding events other than the usual clinical indications.
   (Christian et al. 2004)

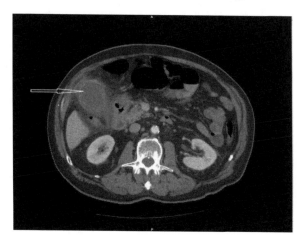

Fig. 4.23 CT scan

206. C – Nausea, vomiting

The common symptoms of the prodromal phase are nausea, vomiting, and diarrhea that occur from minutes to days following exposure. These symptoms may last for minutes up to several days.

(Lombardi 1999)

207. A – Redistribution

(Zaret and Beller 2005)

208. A – Tc-99m thyroid image is subtracted from Tl-201 parathyroid image

Residual activity in the "subtraction" image represents activity in the abnormal parathyroid tissue.

(Palestro 2005)

209. A – 56 mCi

Decay initial given activity of 250 mCi at 7:00 a.m. to 9:00 a.m. and subtract 20 mCi. Use answer obtained from 9:00 A.M. decay/subtraction to get answer for 11:00 A.M. Follow the same process to obtain answer for 3:00 P.M.

(Appendix A, Formula 25)

210. A – The right median basilic vein

The injection technique is a important part of the first pass study and can be given via the external jugular vein or through the median basilic vein in the right arm which provides the most direct path to the right heart.

(Zaret and Beller 2005)

211. C – Bed rest
    (Cohn 2006)

212. C – Whole-body radioiodine scanning and serum thyroglobulin level
    The use of both techniques together is superior than using either one alone.
    (Krausz 2001)

213. A – Convert CT image values to PET attenuation coefficients
    The attenuation correction factor depends on the energy of the photons
    ~70 keV CT X-ray photons must be scaled to the 511 keV PET photons.
    (Saha 2005)

214. D – Influx of red blood cells
    Scintigraphic images are based on physiochemic processes in tissues and do
    not depend on structural changes.
    (Boerman et al. 2001)

215. B – Standardized uptake value
    The imaging must take place always at the same late time point, if results are
    to be compared to previous measurements.
    (Lin and Alavi 2009)

216. A – A decrease in blood volume
    The physiologic actions of BNP include decrease in systemic vascular resis-
    tance and central venous pressure as well as an increase in natriuresis – the
    process of excretion of sodium in the urine resulting in decrease in blood vol-
    ume and a decrease in cardiac output. BNP is a part of the body's natural
    defense mechanisms designed to protect the heart from stress.
    (Family Health Guide 2010)

217. C – Iodide
    (Early and Sodee 1995)

218. A – Photoangioplasty
    (Rockson et al. 2000)

219. D – 76%
    (Appendix A, Formula 38B)

220. D – Chronic CAD
    ACS – life threatening disorder covers the spectrum of clinical conditions that
    are a major cause of emergency medical care and hospitalization in the USA.
    (Zaret and Beller 2005)

References and Suggested Readings

AHA. Cardiac procedures and surgeries. http://www.heart.org/HEARTORG/Conditions/HeartAttack/PreventionTreatmentofHeartAttack/Cardiac-Procedures-and-Surgeries_UCM_303939_Article.jsp. Accessed 15 Sept 2010.

Alessi AM, Farrell MB, Grabher JB, et al. Nuclear cardiology study guide. Reston, VA: SNM; 2010.

Andreoli TE, Bennett JC, et al. Cecil essentials of medicine. 5th ed. Philadelphia, PA: WB Saunders Company; 2001.

Bajc M, Neilly B, Miniati M, Mortensen J, Jonson B. Methodology for ventilation/perfusion SPECT. Semin Nucl Med. 2010;40:415–25.

Bleeker-Rovers CP, Van der Meer JWM, Oyen WJG. Fever of unknown origin. Semin Nucl Med. 2009;39:81–7.

Boerman CO, Rennen H, Oyen JGW, Corstens HMF. Radiopharmaceuticals to image infection and inflammation. Semin Nucl Med. 2001;31:286–95.

Braunwald L et al. Harrison's principles of internal medicine. 15th ed. New York, NY: McGraw-Hill, Inc.; 2001.

Brix G, Lechel U, Glatting G, et al. Radiation exposure of patients undergoing whole-body dual-modality F-18 FDG PET/CT examinations. J Nucl Med. 2005;46:608–13.

CDC. Emergency preparadness and response. Glossary. http://www.bt.cdc.gov/radiation/glossary.asp. Accessed 28 Aug 2010.

Chaffins JA. Paget disease of bone. Radiol Technol. 2007;79:27–40.

Christian PE, Bernier DR, Langan JK. Nuclear medicine and PET. Technology and techniques. 5th ed. St. Louis, MO: Mosby; 2004.

ClinicalTrials.gov. Prospective investigation of pulmonary embolism diagnosis III. http://clinical-trials.gov/ct2/show/NCT00241826. Accessed 17 Oct 2010.

Cohn JN. Cardiac remodeling: basic aspects. Official reprint from UpToDate: http://www.uptodate.com. Accessed 19 Apr 2006.

Early PJ, Sodee BD. Principles and practice of nuclear medicine. 2nd ed. St. Louis, MO: Mosby; 1995.

Emedicine. Angiodysplasia of the colon. http://emedicine.medscape.com/article/170719-overview. Accessed 14 Sept 2010.

English RJ, Brown SE. SPECT single photon emission computed tomography: a primer. 2nd ed. New York, NY: The Society of Nuclear Medicine; 1990.

Family Health Guide. Harvard Medical School. http://www.health.harvard.edu/fhg/updates/BNP-An-important-new-cardiac-test.shtml. Accessed 22 Sept 2010.

Ford PV, Bartold SP, Fink-Bennett DM, et al. Procedure guidelines for gastrointestinal bleeding and Meckel's diverticulum scintigraphy. Society of Nuclear Medicine. J Nucl Med. 1999;40:1226–32.

Frohlich ED. Rypin's basic sciences review. 18th ed. Philadelphia, PA: J.B. Lippincott Company; 2001.

GE Healthcare. AdreView™ Iobenguane I 123 injection. Package insert; 2010.

Gnanasegaran G, Gary CG, Adamson K, Fogelman I. Patterns, variants, artifacts, and pitfalls in conventional radionuclide bone imaging and SPECT/CT. Semin Nucl Med. 2009;39:380–95.

Goldsmith SJ. Radioimmunotherapy of lymphoma: Bexxar and Zevalin. Semin Nucl Med. 2010;40:122–35.

Groch MW, Erwin WD. SPECT in the year 2000. Basic principles. J Nucl Med Technol. 2000;4:233–44.

Grünwald F, Ezziddin S. 131I-Metaiodobenzylguanidine therapy of neuroblastoma and other neuroendocrine tumors. Semin Nucl Med. 2010;40:153–63.

Halama RJ. Radiation safety, radiopharmacy, instrumentation and physics. 13th Annual Nuclear Medicine Review Course. Consultants in Nuclear Medicine (2010). 30 Aug to 01 Sept 2010.

HeathImaging.com. Molecular imaging portal. 4D PET/CT edges into clinical practice. http://www.healthimaging.com. Accessed 17 Oct 2010.

Howarth DM. The role of nuclear medicine in the detection of acute gastrointestinal bleeding. Semin Nucl Med. 2006;36:133–46.

Interstroke. Ten modifiable risk factors explain 90% of stroke risk. TheHeart.org http://www.theheart.org/article/1088693.do. Accessed 21 Jun 2010.

Jefferson Lab. Radiation biological effects. http://www.jlab.org/div_dept/train/rad_guide/effects.html. Accessed 19 Aug 2010.

Kassis AI. Therapeutic radionuclides. Biophysical and radiobiologic principles. Semin Nucl Med. 2008;38:358–66.

Krausz Y. Nuclear endocrinology as a monitoring tool. Semin Nucl Med. 2001;31:238–50.

Lin CE, Alavi A. PET and PET/CT. A clinical guide. 2nd ed. New York, NY: Thieme; 2009.

Lombardi MH. Radiation safety in nuclear medicine. Boca Raton, FL: CRC Press LLC; 1999.

Love C, Palestro CJ. Altered biodistribution and incidental findings on gallium and labeled leukocyte/bone marrow scans. Semin Nucl Med. 2010;40(4):271–82.

Medicare reimbursement for positron emission tomography (PET) procedures. http://www.gehealthcare.com/usen/community/reimbursement/docs/PEToverview.pdf. Accessed 2 Oct 2010.

Medical Physics Consultants, Inc. http://mpcphysics.com/documents/hazmatDOTworkbook10.09.pdf. Accessed 31 Oct 2010.

Medscape Radiology. CT and radiation. http://www.medscape.com/viewarticle/572551_4. Accessed 20 June 2010.

Medscape Radiology. Radiation imaging: slideshow. http://www.medscape.com/features/slideshow/radiation-imaging?src=ptalk&uac=94641PJ. Accessed 20 June 2010.

Mettler FA, Guiberteau MJ. Essentials of nuclear medicine imaging. 5th ed. Philadelphia, PA: Saunders Elsevier; 2006.

Mettler FA, Bhargavan M, et al. Nuclear medicine exposure in the United States, 2005–2007: preliminary results. Semin Nucl Med. 2008;38(5):384–91.

Mycek MJ, Harvey RA. Lippincott's illustrated reviews: pharmacology. 3rd ed. Philadelphia, PA: Lippincott; 2008.

NCRP Composite Glossary. http://www.ncrponline.org/PDFs/NCRP%20Composite%20Glossary.pdf. Accessed 04 Sept 2010.

NRC. Biological effects of radiation. http://www.nrc.gov/reading-rm/basic-ref/teachers/09.pdf. Accessed 19 Aug 2010.

Nuclear Medicine Tutorials. http://www.nucmedtutorials.com/dwnrc/nrc2-1.html. Accessed 7 June 2010.

O'Connor MK, Kemp BJ. Single-photon emission computed tomography/computed tomography: basic instrumentation and innovations. Semin Nucl Med. 2006;36:258–66.

Odunsi ST, Camilleri M. Selected interventions in nuclear medicine: gastrointestinal motor functions. Semin Nucl Med. 2009;39:186–94.

Palestro JC, Tomas BM, Tronco GG. Radionuclide imaging of the parathyroid glands. Semin Nucl Med. 2005;35:266–76.

Perry AG, Potter PA. Clinical nursing skills and techniques. 7th ed. St. Louis, MO: Mosby Elsevier; 2006.

PIOPED III. In: Journal of Thoracic Imaging. Results Summary by Paul Stein and Pam Woodard. http://journals.lww.com/thoracicimaging/blog/JTIBlog/pages/post.aspx?PostID=16. Accessed 27 Sept 2010.

Pitman KT. Sentinel node localization in head and neck tumors. Semin Nucl Med. 2005;35:253–6.

Podrid PJ. ECG tutorial. Official reprint from UpToDate. http://www.uptodate.com. Accessed 05 May 2008.

Radiologyinfo.com. Radiation exposure in X-ray and CT examinations. http://www.radiologyinfo.org/. Accessed 24 Sept 2010.

Rockson SG, Kramer P, et al. Photoangioplasty for human peripheral atherosclerosis. Circulation. 2000;102:2322.

Saha GB. Fundamentals of nuclear pharmacy. 5th ed. New York, NY: Springer; 2004.

Saha GB. Basics of PET imaging. New York, NY: Springer; 2005.

Saha GB. Physics and radiobiology of nuclear medicine. 3rd ed. New York, NY: Springer; 2006.

Sarkar SD. Benign thyroid disease: what is the role of nuclear medicine? Semin Nucl Med. 2006;36:185–93.

Sathekge M. The potential role of Ga-68 labeled peptides in PET imaging of infection. Nucl Med Commun. 2008;29:663–5.

Sircar S. Principles of medical physiology. New York, NY: Thieme; 2008.

Smith J, Oates E. Radionuclide imaging of the thyroid gland: patterns, pearls, and pitfalls. Clin Nucl Med. 2004;29:181–93.

SNM. Procedure guideline for therapy of thyroid disease with iodine-131. J Nucl Med. 2002;43(6):856–61.

Soret M, Bacharach SL, Buvat I. Partial-volume effect in PET tumor imaging. J Nucl Med. 2007;48:932–45.

Springer. Radioactive decay and interaction of radiation with matter. http://www.springer.com/cda/content/document/cda_downloaddocument/9781441908049-c1.pdf. Accessed 26 Sept 2010.

Stein PD, Woodard PK, Weg JG, et al. Diagnostic pathways in acute pulmonary embolism: recommendations of the PIOPED II investigators. Radiology. 2007;242:15–21.

The FreeDictionary. Accessed 17 Sept 2010.

Thyrogen. http://www.thyrogen.com/healthcare/about/thy_hc_clinical_pharmacology.asp. Accessed 27 Sept 2010

U.S. Department of Health and Human Services. REMM. http://www.remm.nlm.gov/effective-dose_definition.htm. Accessed 04 Sept 2010.

U.S. Environmental Protection Agency. Radiation Glossary. http://www.epa.gov/rpdweb00/rert/radfacts.html. Accessed 23 Sept 2010.

U.S. NRC. Transportation of radioactive materials. http://www.nrc.gov/reading-rm/basic-ref/teachers/unit5.html. Accessed 17 Oct 2010.

Vallabhajosula S, Killeen R, Osborne J. Altered biodistribution of radiopharmaceuticals: role of radiochemical/pharmaceutical purity, physiological, and pharmacologic factors. Semin Nucl Med. 2010;40:220–41.

Wahl RL. Principles and practice of PET and PET/CT. 2nd ed. Philadelphia, PA: Lippincott and Wilkins; 2009.

Wikipedia. Basic physics of nuclear medicine/computers in nuclear medicine. http://en.wikipedia.org/wiki. Accessed 19 June 2010.

Wikipedia. http://en.wikipedia.org/wiki. Accessed 2010.

Zanzonico P. Routine quality control of clinical nuclear medicine instrumentation: a brief review. J Nucl Med. 2008;49:1114–31.

Zaret BL, Beller GA. Clinical nuclear cardiology: state of the art and future directions. 3rd ed. Philadelphia, PA: Mosby; 2005.

Ziessman H. Interventions used with cholescintigraphy for the diagnosis of hepatobiliary disease. Semin Nucl Med. 2009;39:174–85.

Zuckier LS, Kolano J. Radionuclide studies in the determination of brain death: criteria, concepts, and controversies. Semin Nucl Med. 2008;38:262–73.

Appendix A
Numbers, Formulas, and Normal Range of Values

Numbers

1. Radiation Safety

The table below describes common radiation exposure limits.

Occupational exposure limits	
Whole body	5 rem (50 mSv)/year
Skin or any extremity	50 rem (500 mSv)/year
Any organ or tissue	50 rem (500 mSv)/year
Lens of eye	15 rem (150 mSv)/year
Fetus of radiation worker	0.5 rem (5 mSv)/year
General public exposure limits	
Whole body	0.1 rem (1 mSv)/year

Steves and Wells (2004)

2. Department of Transportation (DOT) Labels

Department of Transportation regulates the shipment of the radioactive materials; therefore, appropriate labels must be affixed to radioactive shipment packages.

Class	Exposure rate at the package surface cannot exceed (mR/h)	Exposure rate at 1 m from the package cannot exceed (mR/h)
Radioactive I (white)	0.5	No detectable radiation
Radioactive II (yellow)	50	1
Radioactive III (yellow)	200	10

Steves and Wells (2004)

A. Moniuszko and D. Patel, *Nuclear Medicine Technology Study Guide: A Technologist's Review for Passing Board Exams*, DOI 10.1007/978-1-4419-9362-5, © Springer Science+Business Media, LLC 2011

3. Radiation Signs

- **Caution: Radioactive Materials**
  - Posted in area where radioactive materials are stored and exceed the limit of 2 mR/h (millirem per hour) or 0.02 mSv/h (millisievert per hour)
- **Caution: Radiation Area**
  - Posted where one can receive more than 5 mR/h (0.05 mSv) at 30 centimeters (cm)
- **Caution: High Radiation Area**
  - Posted where one can receive more than 100 mR/h (1 mSv) at 30 cm
- **Grave Danger: Very High Radiation Area**
  - Posted in the front of area where one can receive more than 500 rads (5 grays) in 1 h at 1 m from the radiation source

Steves and Wells (2004)

4. Radiopharmacy

- **Reactor produced isotopes:**
  - Mo-99/Tc-99m, I-131, I-125, Xe-133, Cr-51, Sr-89, Sm-153, and P-32
- **Accelerator produced radionuclides:**
  - I-123, Ga-67, Tl-201, In-111, and all positron emitters
- **Molybdenum limits per millicurie of technetium:**
  - Amount of Mo-99 (molybdenum) per mCi (millicurie) of Tc-99m (Technetium) allowed is ≤0.15 mCi (microcurie)
- **MAA particles:**
  - Size of the MAA particles should be 10–90 μm and recommended particles for adult dose is 200,000–700,000
- **Sulfur colloid particles:**
  - Sulfur colloid particles for the liver–spleen scan should be at size 0.01–1 μm

Steves and Wells (2004)

5. Half-Life and Energy of Radioisotopes

Half-life and energy of the commonly used radioisotopes are critical and should be memorized for the exam.

Isotope	Half-life	Energy (keV, kiloelectron volt)
Tc-99m	6 h	140
Tl-201	73 h	68, 81
In-111	2.83 days	173, 247
Xe-133	5.3 days	81
F-18	110 min	511
Co-57	270 days	122
I-123	13.2 h	159
I-125	60 days	35
I-131	8 days	365
Ga-67	78 h	92, 184, 300

Steves and Wells (2004)

Positron emitters

Isotope	Half-life
Rb-82	75 s
O-15	2.1 min
N-13	9 min
C11	20 min
F-18	110 min

Christian et al. (2004)

6. Decay Scheme

The table below describes the decay scheme with arrow and the change in atomic number (Z) during the decay process.

Schemes of decay	Arrow description	Atomic number change(Z)
Alpha (α)	Arrow going downward left	Decreased by two (−2)
Beta (ß⁻)	Arrow going downward right	Atomic number increased by one (+1)
Beta (ß⁺) (positron)	Arrow going downward left	Decreased by one (−1)
Electron capture (EC)	Arrow going downward left	Decreased by one (−1)
Gamma emission (γ)	Arrow going downward straight	No change in atomic number

Christian et al. (2004)

7. Quality Control of Dose Calibrator

The quality control of dose calibrator, type of the test, frequency, and description of tests are given in the following table.

Type of test[a]	Rate of recurrence	Reason of the test
Constancy	Daily before use	To check the reproducibility of dose calibrator by the source of the known activity from day to day
Linearity	Quarterly	To check the ability of dose calibrator to measure the wide range of activity from millicurie (mCi) to microcurie (µCi) amounts
Accuracy	Annually	To check the ability of dose calibrator to measure the different levels of gamma energy (100–500 keV)
Geometry	At installation	Test for the measurement of activity as the volume of radioactive source changes

Steves and Wells (2004)

[a] All tests should be performed after installation of the new equipment, after adjustment, and after repair

8. Quality Control of Scintillation Camera

Quality control of scintillation camera varies upon camera manufactures' recommendation. The following table describes the tests, frequency of occurrence, and reason for the test.

Type of test[a]	Frequency of the test	Description
Field uniformity	Daily	Ability of the detector to produce uniform image when source provides uniform photon distribution
Spatial resolution	Weekly	Ability of the detector to distinguish small objects in space
Spatial linearity	Weekly	Ability of the detector to depict true straight line, corresponding straight line in phantom (actual depiction of true organ)
SPECT center of rotation (COR)	Weekly or monthly	Used to correct slight variation in the detector position as it rotates

Steves and Wells (2004)

[a] These tests should be performed after repair or preventative maintenance

Testing frequencies are recommended by the camera manufacturer

9. Unit Conversions

A. Conversion from Ci (curie) to mCi (millicurie) to μCi (microcurie), and GBq (gigabecquerel) to MBq (megabecquerel) to kBq (kilobecquerel)
- 1 Ci = 1,000 mCi = 1,000,000 μCi
- 1 GBq = 1,000 MBq = 1,000,000 kBq

B. Conversion between Ci and GBq
- 1 Ci = 37 GBq = 37,000 MBq = 37,000,000 kBq
- 1 GBq = 0.027 Ci or 27 mCi or 27,000 μCi
- 1 Bq = 2.7×10^{-11} Ci

C. Conversion between rad (radiation absorbed dose) and gray (Gy)
- 1 Gy = 100 rad = 10,000 mrad
- 1 rad = 0.01 Gy = 0.0001 mGy

D. Conversion of Sievert and rem (roentgen equivalent in man)
- 1 Sv = 100 rem
- 1 rem = 0.01 Sv

E. Conversion between pound and kilogram
- 1 lb = 0.45 kg
- 1 kg = 2.2 lb

F. Conversion of length
- 1 ft = 12 in. = 30.5 cm

Wells and Martha (1999)

Formulas

10. Calculation of Percent Error or Percent Difference

A. Percentage error or percentage difference

- Percent error or percent difference $= \dfrac{\text{Expected} - \text{Actual}}{\text{Expected}} \times 100\%$

B. Correction factor

- Correction factor $= \dfrac{\text{Expected activity}}{\text{Actual activity}}$

Wells and Martha (1999)

11. Net Counts

Net counts = Gross counts − Background counts

Wells and Martha (1999)

12. Standard Deviation of Series of Values

- $SD = \sqrt{\dfrac{\sum (n-\bar{n})^2}{N-1}}$

  - Σ = symbol of sum, meaning value following this needs to be summed
  - $\text{Mean} = \dfrac{\text{Sum of all values}}{\text{Total number of values}}$
  - $\bar{n}$ = mean of value
  - n = individual value
  - N = total number of values

13. Standard Deviation for a Single Value

- CI = confidence interval
- n = the single value
- 68% confidence interval (±1 standard deviation):
  $CI_{68\%} = n \pm \sqrt{n}$ or $CI_{68\%} = n \pm 1\ SD$
- 95% confidence interval (±2 standard deviation):
  $CI_{95\%} = n \pm 2\sqrt{n}$ or $CI_{95\%} = n \pm 2\ SD$
- 99% confidence interval (±3 standard deviation):
  $CI_{99\%} = n \pm 3\sqrt{n}$ or $CI_{99\%} = n \pm 3\ SD$

Wells and Martha (1999)

14. Percentage Error of Single Value or ($\%$SD)

Standard deviation or confidence interval

- $\%68\ SD = \dfrac{100\%}{\sqrt{N}}$

- $\%95\ SD = \dfrac{(2)\ (100\%)}{\sqrt{N}}$

- $\%99\ SD = \dfrac{(3)\ (100\%)}{\sqrt{N}}$

Wells and Martha (1999)

[a] Use these above formulas to calculate minimum counts required to determine % error at a given confidence level. Where (N) = number of counts. The level most commonly used in nuclear medicine is 95% Wells and Martha (1999)

15. How to Convert Counts Per Minute (cpm) to Disintegration Per Minute (dpm) Using Well Counter Efficiency

- $dpm = \dfrac{\text{Gross cpm} - \text{Background cpm}}{\text{Efficiency expressed as decimal}}$
  - Simply convert given efficiency in % to decimal, dividing by 100

Wells and Martha (1999)

16. Inverse Square Law

- $(I_1)(D_1)^2 = (I_2)(D_2)^2$
  - I_1 = intensity at original distance D_1
  - I_2 = intensity at newer distance D_2

Wells and Martha (1999)

17. How to Calculate Change in Exposure Rate due to Shielding

- $I = I_0 e^{-(0.693)(x/HVL)}$
  - I = exposure rate being calculated
  - I_0 = original exposure rate
  - e = 2.718 constant know as Euler's number
  - x = thickness of the shielding material
  - HVL = half-value layer for a given shielding material

Wells and Martha (1999)

18. Effective Half-Life

- $T_e = \dfrac{T_P \times T_b}{T_P + T_b}$
  - T_e = effective half-life
  - T_p = physical half-life
  - T_b = biological half-life

Wells and Martha (1999)

19. Energy Resolution (Full-Width at Half-Maximum)

- % Energy resolution $= \dfrac{\text{FWHM in keV}}{\text{Energy of radionuclide in keV}} \times 100\%$

  - Half maximum $= \dfrac{\text{Maximum counts}}{2}$

  - FWHM $=$ Upper limits $-$ Lower limits in keV

Wells and Martha (1999)

20. Chi-Square Value

- $\chi^2 = \dfrac{\sum (n-\bar{n})^2}{n}$

  - $\chi^2 =$ chi-square
  - $n =$ individual values
  - $\bar{n} =$ mean value
  - $N =$ number of value used
  - SD $=$ standard deviation
  - Degree of freedom $= N - 1$ where $N =$ number of values used

Wells and Martha (1999)

21. Well Counter Efficiency

- % Efficiency $= \dfrac{\text{Counts per unit of time (cpm or cps)}}{(\text{Disintegration per unit time})(\text{Mean number per disintegration})} \times 100\%$

Wells and Martha (1999)

22. How to Calculate Energy Window for Pulse Height Analyzer and Percentage Dose Range

A. Energy window
- Energies within windows $=$ Energy in keV $\pm$
  $\dfrac{\text{Energy in keV} \times \text{Percentage window as decimal}}{2}$

B. Acceptable dose range
- Acceptable dose range $=$ dose amount $\pm$ dose amount $\times$ percentage as decimal

Wells and Martha (1999)

23. Gamma-Camera Sensitivity

- Sensitivity as $cpm/\mu Ci = \dfrac{Source\ cpm - Background\ cpm}{Source\ activity\ in\ \mu Ci}$

Wells and Martha (1999)

24. Calculation of Total Memory Used

- Total memory required $= (pixel\ height) \times (pixel\ width) \times (frames)$
  - If study is acquired in byte mode but stored in word mode, then multiply the total memory required (answer from the above formula) with 0.5
  - If study is acquired in word mode but stored in byte mode, then multiply the total memory required (answer from the above formula) with 2

Wells and Martha (1999)

25. Decay Calculation Using Half-Life

- $A_t = A_0 e^{-0.693 \times (t|t_{1/2})}$
  - At = activity at specific time
  - A_0 = original activity
  - e = Euler's number (2.718) which remains constant in equation
  - t = elapsed time
  - $t_{1/2}$ = half-life
- **Use the same formula for precalibration**
  - At = activity at time t (calibration time)
  - A_0 = activity at time 0 (precalibration time)

Wells and Martha (1999)

26. Calculate Activity Using Decay Factor (DF)

- $At = A_0 \times DF$
- At = activity at specific time t
- A_0 = original activity
- DF = decay factor, which is obtained by $e^{-0.693 \times (t|t_{1/2})}$

Wells and Martha (1999)

27. Calculating Activity Using Precalibration Factor

- $At = A_0 \times$ Precalibration factor
- $At =$ activity at time t (calibration time)
- $A_0 =$ activity at time 0 (precalibration time)
- Using decay factor to precalibrate activity $A_0 = \dfrac{A_t}{DF}$ will obtain a same result

Wells and Martha (1999)

28. How to Obtain Concentration and Specific Activity

A. Specific concentration
- Specific concentration $= \dfrac{\text{Activity}}{\text{Volume}}$

B. Specific activity
- Specific activity $=$ Concentration $\times$ Volume

Wells and Martha (1999)

29. How to Calculate Specific Volume

- Volume $= \dfrac{\text{Activity desired}}{\text{Specific concentration}}$ or $\dfrac{\text{What you want}}{\text{What you have}}$

Wells and Martha (1999)

30. How to Calculate Mo-99 Limits, Mo-99 Concentration Per Particular Tc-99m Activity, and Elute or Kit Expiration Time Based on Mo-99 Activity

A. Mo-99 limits
- $X\,\mu Ci$ Mo-99 $= (0.15\ \mu Ci$ Mo-99/mCi Tc-99m)(Tc-99m activity in mCi)

B. Concentration of Mo-99
- $0.15\mu Ci\,$Mo-99$/$mCi Tc - 99m $= \dfrac{\text{Mo - 99 in } \mu Ci}{\text{Tc - 99m in mCi}}$

C. Tc-99m elute or kit expiration time based on Mo-99 activity
- $t = \dfrac{-\ln \text{Mo}_0 / \text{Tc}_0}{0.1052} - 18.03$
- $\text{Mo}_0 =$ initial Mo activity in μCi
- $\text{Tc}_0 =$ initial Tc-99m activity

Wells and Martha (1999)

31. Pediatric Dose Calculation

A. Clark's formula (weight)

- Clark's formula $= \dfrac{(\text{Child's weight in lb})(\text{Adult dose})}{150 \text{ lb}}$

B. Webster's formula (age)

- Webster's formula $= \dfrac{\text{Age (years)} + 1}{\text{Age} + 7} \times \text{Adult dosage}$

C. Young's formula (age)

- Young's formula $= \dfrac{\text{Age (years)}}{\text{Age} + 12} \times \text{Adult dosage}$

Steves and Wells (2004)

32. How to Calculate Percent Radiochemical Purity of Radiopharmaceutical

A. % Purity

- % Purity $= \dfrac{\text{Activity in desired form}}{\text{Total activity}} \times 100\%$

B. % Impurity

- % Impurity $= \dfrac{\text{Activity in undesirable form}}{\text{Total activity}} \times 100\%$

Wells and Martha (1999)

33. How to Calculate Left Ventricle Ejection Fraction

- % EF $= \dfrac{(\text{End - diastolic}) - (\text{End - systolic})}{(\text{End - diastolic})} \times 100\%$

- Net ROI counts = ROI counts $- \left\{ \dfrac{\text{Background ROI counts}}{\text{Background ROI pixel}} \times \text{ROI pixel} \right\}$

Wells and Martha (1999)

34. How to Calculate Gall Bladder Ejection Fraction

- %GBEF $= \dfrac{\text{Net maximum GB counts} - \text{Net minimum GB counts}}{\text{Net maximum GB counts}} \times 100\%$

- Net ROI counts are derived by above Net ROI counts (Formula 33).

Wells and Martha (1999)

35. How to Calculate Gastric Emptying Time

- Geometric mean = $\sqrt{\text{Anterior ROI counts} \times \text{Posterior ROI counts}}$

  A. % Activity *remaining* at time *T*

- % Activity *remaining* at time $T = \dfrac{\text{Geometric mean at time } T}{\text{Geometric mean at time } 0 \times \text{Decay factor for time } T} \times 100\%$

  B. % Activity *emptying* at time *T*

- % Activity *emptying* at time $T = \dfrac{\text{Geometric mean at time } 0 - \text{Geometric mean at time } T}{\text{Geometric mean at time } 0} \times 100\%$

Wells and Martha (1999)

36. Calculation for Voiding Cystogram

A. Expected bladder capacity

- Expected bladder capacity $= (\text{Age} + 2)\,(30\text{ ml})$

B. Calculating residual bladder volume

- Residual bladder volume $= \dfrac{(\text{Voided volume})(\text{Postvoid counts})}{\text{Pre-void couts} - \text{Post-void counts}}$

C. To calculate the actual volume of refluxed urine

- Reflux volume = Reflux ROI counts $\times \dfrac{\text{Total bladder volume}}{\text{Pre-void bladder ROI counts}}$

Wells and Martha (1999)

37. Lung Quantitation

- How to calculate % activity in particular ROI
- % Activity in ROI $= \dfrac{\text{Counts ROI}}{\text{Total counts in all ROI}} \times 100\%$
- *Note*: This formula could be used to calculate percent function or percent uptake in one ROI, when compared to other ROIs

Wells and Martha (1999)

38. How to Calculate Thyroid Uptake

A. Calculating thyroid uptake using identical capsules as standard

- % Uptake $= \dfrac{\text{Thyroid counts} - \text{Thigh counts}}{\text{Capsule counts} - \text{Background}} \times 100\%$

B. Calculating thyroid uptake using patient's capsule for a standard

- % Uptake $= \dfrac{\text{Thyroid counts} - \text{Thigh counts}}{(\text{Capsule counts} - \text{Background})(\text{Decay factor})} \times 100\%$

Wells and Martha (1999)

39. How to Prepare Dilute Solution from Stock Solution

- $C_1 V_1 = C_2 V_2$
- C_1 = original concentration or stock concentration
- V_1 = original volume
- C_2 = final concentration
- V_2 = final volume

Wells and Martha (1999)

Normal Range of Values

40. Esophageal Transit Time

- Transit rates >90% after one to eight swallows
- 4% of the maximal esophageal activity by 10 min

Shackett (2008)

41. Gastric Emptying

- Normal values for low-fat, egg-white gastric emptying scintigraphy.

Time	Lower normal limit gastric retention (%)	Upper normal limit gastric retention (%)
0 min		
0.5 h	70	
1.0 h	30	90
2.0 h		60
3.0 h		30
4.0 h		10

Abell et al. (2010)
- These values are the 95th percentile confidence interval.
- A lower value suggests rapid gastric emptying.
- A greater value suggests delayed gastric emptying.

42. GBEF

- 24–95% at 60 min in healthy subjects by half-and-half milk
- 33% at 60 min using a lactose-free food supplement
- Between 35 and 75% using cholecystokinin (CCK)
- Different results in different studies may be due to: a different fatty meal and different methodology, e.g., different CCK infusion time

Ziessman (2009)

43. LVEF

- LVEF at rest: $62.3 \pm 6.1\%$ (1 SD) with a lower limit of normal of 50%
- RVEF at rest: $52.3 \pm 6.2\%$ ($N = 365$) with a lower limit of normal of 40%
- Weighted mean normal values assessed by radionuclide angiocardiography

Zaret and Beller (2005)

44. LVEF

	Typical	Normal range
EDV (ml)	120	65–240
ESV (ml)	50	16–143
EF (%)	58	55–70

Wikipedia (2010)

45. Tc-99m MAG3 Renography: Normal Values

- **Kidney**
  - % Uptake: 42–58%
  - T max. (min): 2.1–6.3
  - Time to half max (min): 3.5–8.3
  - 20 min cts/max: 0.12–0.54
- **Cortical**
  - Time to peak (min): 2.1–3.6
  - Time to half max (min): 3.2–8.8
  - 20 min cts/max: 0.12–0.34

Esteves et al. (2006)

46. RCM

(a) Widely accepted upper limits for the normal range are:
  - 36 ml/kg in adult males[a]
  - 32 ml/kg in adult females[a]

Early and Sodee (1995)
[a] These values are appropriate for persons who are not overweight

47. Thyroid

- Serum Triiodothyronine T3: −80 to 180 ng/dl
- Serum thyrotropin TSH: −0.5 to 6 U/ml
- Serum thyroglobulin Tg: 0–30 ng/m

48. Normal Range Values of Radioactive Iodine Uptake (RAIU)

- 6 h: 6–18%
- 24 h: 10–35%

Note: Values may vary depending on the amount of iodine in patient diet, standards, variety of equipment, etc. and normal value ranges may vary slightly among different laboratories
Society of Nuclear Medicine (2010)

References and Suggested Readings

Abell TL, Camilleri M, Donohoe K, Hasler WL, Lin HC, Alan H, et al. Consensus recommendations for gastric emptying scintigraphy: a joint report of the American Neurogastroenterology and Motility Society and the Society of Nuclear Medicine. J Nucl Med Technol. 2008;36(1): 44–54. http://tech.snmjournals.org/cgi/rapidpdf/jnmt.107.048116v1. Accessed 16 Nov 2010.

Christian PE, Bernier DR, Langan JK. Nuclear medicine and PET. Technology and techniques. 5th ed. St. Louis, MO: Mosby; 2004.

Early PJ, Sodee DB. Principles and practices of nuclear medicine. 2nd ed. St. Louis, MO: Mosby; 1995.

Esteves PF, Taylor A, Manatunga A, Russell D, Folks DR, Krishnan M, et al. Tc-99m MAG3 renography: normal values for MAG3 clearance and curve parameters, excretory parameters, and residual urine volume. Am J Roentgenol. 2006;187:W610–7.

Shackett P. Nuclear medicine technology: procedure and quick reference. 2nd ed. Philadelphia, PA: Lippincott Williams & Wilkins; 2008.

Society of Nuclear Medicine. Society of Nuclear Medicine procedure guideline for thyroid uptake measurement. http://www.nucmedinfo.com/pdf/guidelines/Thyroid%20Uptake%20 Measurement.pdf. Accessed 16 Nov 2010.

Steves AM, Wells AM. Review of nuclear medicine technology: preparation for certification examinations. Reston, VA: Society of Nuclear Medicine; 2004.

Wells P, Martha P. Practical mathematics in nuclear medicine technology. Reston, VA: Society of Nuclear Medicine; 1999.

Wikipedia. Ejection fraction. http://en.wikipedia.org/wiki/Ejection_fraction. Accessed 16 Nov 2010.

Zaret BL, Beller GA. Clinical nuclear cardiology: state of the art and future directions. 3rd ed. Philadelphia, PA: Mosby; 2005.

Ziessman H. Interventions used with cholescintigraphy for the diagnosis of hepatobiliary disease. Semin Nucl Med. 2009;39:174–85.

Appendix B
Commonly Used Abbreviations and Symbols in Nuclear Medicine

Abbreviations

AAA	Abdominal aortic aneurysm
ABC	Airway, breathing, circulation
ABG	Arterial blood gases
ABW	Adjusted body weight
A/C	Assist control ventilation
ACD	Acid-citrate-dextrose
ACE	Angiotensin-converting enzyme
ACLS	Advance cardiac life support
ACS	Acute coronary syndrome
ACTH	Adrenocorticotropic hormone
ADC	Analog-to-digital converter
ADL	Activities of daily living
AED	Automated external defibrillator
AF	Atrial fibrillation
AFB	Acid fast bacilli
AFL	Atrial flutter
AICD	Automatic implantable cardiac defibrillator
AIDS	Acquired immune deficiency syndrome
AKA	Above knee amputation
ALS	Advance life support
AMA	Against medical advice
AMI	Acute myocardial infarction
AMV	Assisted mechanical ventilation
Angio.	Angiogram; angiography
AO	Aorta

APC	Atrial premature contraction
Approx.	Approximately; approximated
ARB	Angiotensin receptor blocker
ARC	AIDS-related complex
ARDS	Adult respiratory distress syndrome
ARF	Acute renal failure
ARS	Acute radiation syndrome
ASA	Acetylsalicylic acid (Aspirin)
ASAP	As soon as possible
ATN	Acute tubular necrosis
AV	Arteriovenous
A-V	Arterioventricular
AVM	Arteriovenous malformation
AVN	Avascular necrosis
AVR	Aortic valve replacement
Ax	Axilla, axillary
BASIC	Beginner's all-purpose symbolic instruction code
BBB	Bundle branch block
BBB	Blood–brain barrier
BE	Barium enema
BG	Blood glucose
BID	Twice daily
Bil	Bilateral
BLS	Basic life support
BM	Bowel movement
BMI	Body mass index
BNP	Brain natriuretic peptide
BP	Blood pressure
BPH	Benign prostatic hypertrophy
Bpm	Beats per minute
BRADY	Bradycardia
BRBPR	Bright red blood per rectum
BSA	Body surface area
BUN	Blood urea nitrogen
Bx	Biopsy
CA	Cancer, carcinoma
CABG	Coronary artery bypass graft
CACS	Coronary artery calcium score
CAD	Coronary artery disease
CAP	Community acquired pneumonia
Cath	Catheterization

CBC	Complete blood count
CBD	Common bile duct
CBF	Cerebral blood flow
CCK	Cholecystokinin
CCT	Cardiac computed tomography
CCTA	Cardiac computed tomographic angiography
C. diff	Clostridium difficile
CE	Cardiac enzymes
CEA	Carcinoembryonic antigen
CHF	Congestive heart failure
Chol	Cholesterol
Chr	Chronic
CK-MB	Creatine kinase-myocardial band
cm	Centimeter
CMR	Cardiac magnetic resonance
CNA	Certified nursing assistant
CO	Cardiac output
CO_2	Carbon dioxide
COPD	Chronic obstructive pulmonary disease
COR	Center of rotation
COTA	Certified occupation therapy assistant
CP	Chest pain
CPR	Cardiopulmonary resuscitation
CPT	Current procedural terminology
CPU	Central processing unit
CRF	Chronic renal failure
CRP	C-Reactive protein
CSF	Cerebrospinal fluid
CT	Computerized tomography
CVA	Cerebrovascular accident
CVD	Cardiovascular disease
DAC	Digital-to-analog converter
D/C	Discharge
Decub.	Decubitus
DEXA	Dual-energy X-ray absorptiometry
DIC	Disseminated intravascular coagulation
DICOM	Digital imaging and communications in medicine
DJD	Degenerative joint disease
DM	Diabetes mellitus
DMA	Direct memory access
DMSA	Dimercaptosuccinic acid
DNA	Deoxyribonucleic acid

DNR	Do not resuscitate
D. O.	Doctor of osteopathy
DOA	Dead on arrival
DOB	Date of birth
DOE	Dyspnea on exertion
dpm	Disintegrations per minute
DRE	Digital rectal examination
DTPA	Diethylene triamine pentaacetic acid
DTPI	Dual time-point imaging
DUI	Driving under the influence
DVT	Deep venous thrombosis
Dx	Diagnosis
e.g.	For example
E. S.R.D.	End stage renal disease
Ea.	Each
EBL	Estimated blood loss
ECG	Electrocardiogram
EENT	Eye, ear, nose, and throat
ED	End diastole
EF	Ejection fraction
EGD	EsophagoGastroDuodenoscopy
EMG	ElectroMyography
EP	Electrophysiology
Eq	Equal
ERCP	Endoscopic retrograde cholangiography
ERNA	Equilibrium radionuclide angiography
ES	End systole
ESBLs	Extended spectrum betalactamases
ESR	Erythocyte sedimentation rate
et	And
ET	Emory toolbox
Etc	Et cetera
ETOH	Ethyl alcohol
Eval	Evaluation
Excl.	Exclude
Exp.	Expired
Extr.	Extremities
FBP	Filtered back projection
FBS	Fasting blood sugar
FDG	FluoroDeoxyGlucose
Fluoro	Fluoroscopy

FN	False negative
FNA	Fine needle aspiration
Ft	Feet (length)
FIT	Failure to thrive
FOV	Field of view
FP	False positive
f/u	Follow up
FUO	Fever of unknown origin
Fx	Fracture
GB	Gallbladder
GBEF	Gallbladder ejection fraction
GERD	GastroEsophageal reflux disease
GFR	Glomerular filtration rate
GI	GastroIntestinal
GLU	Glucose
Gm	Gram
G-tube	Gastrostomy tube
H	Hour
HAMA	Human antimouse antibodies
HAP	Hospital acquired pneumonia
Hb	Hemoglobin
HbA1c	Glycosylated hemoglobin
HCG	Human chorionic gonadotropin
Hct	Hematocrit
HCTZ	Hydrochlorothiazide
HD	High definition
HDL	High-density lipoprotein
HDP	Hydroxyethylene diphosphonate
HEENT	Head, eyes, ears, nose, throat
HELLP	Hemolysis, elevated liver enzymes, low platelets
H/H	Hemoglobin/hematocrit
HIDA	Hepatobiliary Imino-diacetic acid, hydroxyiminodiacetic acid
HIV	Human immuodeficiency virus
HMPAO	Hexamethylpropyleneamine oxime
H/O	History of
H&P	History and physical
HR	Heart rate
HRES	High resolution
HRT	Hormone replacement therapy
HTN	Hypertension

IBS	Irritable bowel syndrome
IBW	Ideal body weight
ICCU	Intensive coronary care unit
ICD-9	International classification of diseases (9th revision)
ICU	Intensive care unit
IDDM	Insulin-dependent diabetes mellitus
Ig	Immunoglobin
IHD	Ischemic heart disease
IMP	IodoaMPhetamine
Inc	incontinent
INF	Inferior
Inj	Injection
Insuff	Insufficiency
INT	Interior
I/O	Intake and output
IPAP	Inspiratory positive airway pressure
IQ	Intelligence quotient
ITLC	Instant thin layer chromatography
IV	Intravenous(ly)
IVC	Inferior vena cava
JPEG	Joint photographic experts group
k	Kilo
K	Thousand
Kcal	Kilocalories
KCl	Potassium chloride
keV	Kiloelectronvolts
Kg	Kilogram
KUB	Kidneys, ureters, and bladder X-ray
L	Liter
LA	Left atrium
LAD	Left anterior descending
LAN	Local area network
LBBB	Left bundle branch block
LCA	Left coronary artery
LCX	Left circumflex artery
LDL	Lower density lipoprotein
LE	Lower extremity
LEAP	Low energy, all purpose
LEHR	Low energy, high resolution
LEHS	Low energy, high sensitivity

LET	Linear energy transfer
LFOV	Large field of view
LFT	Liver function tests
LIMA	Left internal mammary artery
LLAT	Left lateral
LLL	Left lower lobe
LLQ	Left lower quadrant
LMA	Left main artery
LMP	Last menstrual period
LPN	Licensed practical nurse
LPO	Left posterior oblique
L-S	Lumbo-sacral
LUE	Left upper extremity
LUL	Left upper lobe
LUQ	Left upper quadrant
LUT	Lookup table
LV	Left ventricle
LVEF	Left ventricle ejection fraction
LVG	Left ventriculography
LVH	Left ventricular hypertrophy
m	Meter
MAA	Macroaggregated albumin
MAG 3	MercaptuAcetyltriGlycine
MBq	MegaBecquerel
MCA	Middle cerebral artery
MCHC	Mean corpuscular hemoglobin concentrate
mCi	Millicurie
MCL	Medial collateral ligament
MCV	Mean corpuscular volume
MDP	Methylene diphosphonate
MEAP	Medium energy, all purpose
mEq	Milliequivalent
MET	Metabolic equivalent of task
mg	Milligram
MHR	Multiple head registration
MI	Myocardial infarction
MIBG	MetaIodoBenzylGuanidine
MIRD	Medical internal radiation dose
μCi	Microcurie
μg	Microgram
MIP	Maximum intensity projection

ml	Milliliter
MLEM	Maximum-likelihood expectation maximization
M&M	Morbidity and mortality
MMAD	Mass median aerodynamic diameter
MoAb	Monoclonal antibody
MPI	Myocardial perfusion imaging
MR	Mitral regurgitation
MRI	Magnetic resonance imaging
MRSA	Methicillin-resistant *Staphylococcus aureus*
msec	Millisecond(s)
MUGA	Multigated acquisition scan
MV	Mitral valve
MVI	Motor vehicle accident
MVP	Mitral valve prolapse
N/A	Nonapplicable
NaCl	Sodium chloride
NC	Nasal cannula
ng	Nanogram(s)
NGT	Nasogastric tube
NHL	Non-Hodgkin's lymphoma
NIDDM	Noninsulin-dependent diabetes mellitus
NKA	No known allergies
NPH	Normal pressure hydrocephalus
NPO	Nothing per oral
NSTEMI	Non-ST-segment elevation myocardial infarction
NSR	Normal sinus rhythm
N&T	Nose and throat
NTG	Nitroglycerine
N/V/D	Nausea/vomiting/diarrhea
ODS	One day surgery
OOB	Out of bed
OSEM	Ordered subsets expectation maximization
OT	Occupational therapy
OTC	Over the counter
p	After
P	P wave
PA	Pulmonary artery
PAC	Premature atrial contraction
PACS	Picture archiving and communication systems
PCN	Penicillin

PE	Pulmonary embolism
PEG	Percutaneous endoscopic gastrostomy
PET	Positron emission tomography
PET/CT	Positron emission tomography/computed tomography
PFT	Pulmonary function tests
PH	Pulmonary hypertension
pH	Degree of acidity or alkalinity
PICC	Peripherally inserted central catheter
PIOPED	Prospective investigation of pulmonary embolism diagnosis
PMH	Past medical history
PMTs	Photomultiplier tubes
PN	Parenteral nutrition
PNS	Peripheral nervous system
PO	Per os
PRN	As needed
Prox	Proximal
PSA	Prostatic specific antigen
PT	Physical therapy
PTCA	Percutaneous transluminal coronary angioplasty
PVC	Premature ventricular contractions
PVD	Peripheral vascular disease
PVE	Partial-volume effect
PYP	Pyrophosphate
q	Every
QC	Quality control
q.h.	Every hour
q.i.d.	Four times daily
QPS-QGS	Quantitative perfusion SPECT/quantitative gated SPECT
QRS	QRS complex
QS	QS complex
QT	Q to T interval
RA	Right atrium
RAIU	Radioactive iodine uptake
RAM	Random access memory
RAO	Right anterior oblique
RBBB	Right bundle branch block
RBC	Red blood cells
RCA	Right coronary artery
REM	Rapid eye movement
RES	Reticuloendothelial system
RF	Renal failure

Rh	Rhesus blood factor
RIS	Radioimmunoscintigraphy
RISA	Radioactive iodine serum albumin
RLAT	Right lateral
RLE	Right lower extremity
RLL	Right lower lobe
RLQ	Right lower quadrant
RLS	Restless leg syndrome
R/O	Rule out
ROM	Read only memory
RN	Registered nurse
RNA	Radionuclide angiography
RNA	Ribonucleic acid
R/O	Rule out
ROM	Range of motion
RP	Radiopharmaceutical
RR	Respiratory rate
RSC	Radiation safety committee
RSO	Radiation safety officer
RT	Radiation therapy
RUE	Right upper extremity
RUL	Right upper lobe
RUQ	Right upper quadrant
RV	Right ventricle
Rx	Prescription
S1, S2, S3 etc	First sacral, second sacral, third sacral vertebra, etc.
SA	Sinoatrial
SC	Sulfur colloid
SB	Sinus bradycardia
SCA	Sudden cardiac arrest
SCLC	Small cell lung carcinoma
SDS	Same day surgery
SDS	Summed difference (stress-rest perfusion) score
SICU	Surgical intensive care unit
SNM	Society of Nuclear Medicine
SOB	Short of breath
S/P	Status post
SPECT	Single photon emission computed tomography
SRS	Summed rest score
S and S	Signs and symptoms
SSKI	Saturated solution of potassium iodide

SSN	Suprasternal notch
SSS	Summed stress score
SSS	Sick sinus syndrome
ST	Sinus tachycardia
ST	ST segment
Stat	Immediately
STD	Sexually transmitted disease
STEMI	ST-segment elevation myocardial infarction
Strep	Streptococcus
Sup	Supine
SUV	Standardized uptake value
SVC	Superior vena cava
SVT	Supraventricular tachycardia
T	T wave
T3	Triodothyronine
T4	Thyroxine
TB	Tuberculosis
t_b	Biological half-life
TDD	Telecommunications device for the deaf
t_e	Effective half-life
TED	Thrombo embolic deterrent (Ted stockings)
TEE	Transesophageal echocardiogram
TF	Tube feeding
THR	Target heart rate
TIA	Transient ischemic attack
TID	Transient ischemic dilation
t.i.d.	Three times a day
TIFF	Tagged image file format
TLD	Thermoluminescent dosimeter
TMJ	Temporal mandibular joint
TN	True negative
TNM	Tumor nodes metastasis
TOD	Tail on detector
TP	True positive
TPN	Total parenteral nutrition
TPR	Temperature, pulse, respiration
TEE	Transesophageal echocardiography
TRH	Thyrotropin-releasing hormone
TSH	Thyroid-stimulating hormone
TTE	Transthoracic echocardiography
TURP	Transurethral resection of prostate

U/A	Urinalysis
UE	Upper extremity
UGI	Upper gastrointestinal
UTI	Urinary tract infection

VAP	Ventilator associated pneumonia
VDRL	Venereal Disease Research Laboratory (blood test for syphillis)
VF SCA	Ventricular fibrillation sudden cardiac arrest
via	By way of
VMA	Vanillymandelic acid
V-P shunt	Ventriculo-peritoneal shunt
VRE	Vancomycin resistant enterococcus
VS	Vital signs
V-tach	Ventricular tachycardia

WAN	Wide area network
WBC	White blood cell
W/C	Wheelchair
WLCQ	Wackers–Liu circumferential quantification
WPW	Wolff–Parkinson–White syndrome

| XRT | Radiation therapy treatment |

| YTD | Year to date |

Symbols

&	And
@	At
√	Check
↓	Decrease
=	Equal
♀	Female
←	From
>	Greater than
↑	High
↑	Increased
+++	Large amount
<	Less than
↓	Low
↓	Decreased
♂	Male

++	Moderate amount
+	More or less
–	Negative
O	No; null; none; nothing
#	Number
O	Objective findings
+	Positive
1°	Primary
(?)	Questionable
2nd	Secondary; second
2°	Secondary to
2°	Second degree
ĉ	With
ŝ	Without

Appendix C
Useful Web Sites

- ACR (American College of Radiology): http://www.acr.org/
- AHA (American Heart Association): http://www.heart.org/
- Amedeo – The Medical Literature Guide: http://www.amedeo.com/
- American AED/CPR Association: http://www.aedcpr.com/
- ANMS (American Neurogastroenterology and Motility Society): http://www.motilitysociety.org/
- ARRT (American Registry of Radiologic Technologists): https://www.arrt.org/index.html
- ASNC (American Society of Nuclear Cardiology): http://www.asnc.org/
- ASRT (American Society of Radiologic Technologists): https://www.asrt.org/
- AuntMinnie.com: http://www.auntminnie.com/
- Brain Atlas: http://www.med.harvard.edu/AANLIB/home.html
- CDC (Centers for Disease Control): http://www.cdc.gov/
- Consultants in Nuclear Medicine: http://www.nucmedconsultants.com/
- DOT (Department of Transportation): http://www.dot.gov/
- Drugs.com: http://www.drugs.com/
- Emedicine: http://emedicine.medscape.com
- EPA (Environmental Protection Agency): http://www.epa.gov/
- Family Health Guide–Harvard Medical School: http://www.health.harvard.edu/fhg/
- FDA (Food and Drug Administration): http://www.fda.gov/
- GE (General Electric) Healthcare: https://hls.gehealthcare.com/gehc/
- HealthImaging.com: http://www.healthimaging.com/
- HFAP (Healthcare Facilities Accreditation Program): http://www.hfap.org/
- HPS (Health Physics Society): http://www.hps.org/
- IAEA (International Atomic Energy Agency): http://www.iaea.org/
- ICANL (Intersocietal Commission for the Accreditation of Nuclear Medicine Laboratories): http://www.icanl.org/icanl/index.htm
- ICRP (International Commission on Radiological Protection): http://www.icrp.org/
- ICRU (International Commission on Radiation Units): http://www.icru.org/

- IMAIOS E-anatomy: http://www.imaios.com/en/e-Anatomy/
- Internet Journal of Nuclear Medicine:
  http://www.ispub.com/ostia/index.php?xmlFilePath=journals/ijnuc/vol3n1/scan.xml
- JCAHO (Joint Commission on Accreditation of Healthcare Organizations):
  http://www.jointcommission.org/
- Jefferson Lab: http://www.jlab.org/div_dept/train/rad_guide/effects.html
- Mallinckrodt Inst of Radiology WU in St. Louis Teaching File:
  http://gamma.wustl.edu/
- Mallinckrodt Institute of Radiology Cases:
  http://www.radquiz.com/Nucs-Teaching.htm
- MDS Nordion: http://www.mds.nordion.com/
- Medical Physics Dept, Pilgrim Hospital, Lincolnshire, UK:
  http://www.nuclearmedicine.org.uk
- Medscape: http://www.medscape.com/
- Molecular Imaging: http://www.molecularimaging.net/
- NCBI (National Center for Biotechnology Information):
  http://www.ncbi.nlm.nih.gov/pubmed/
- NCI (National Cancer Institute): http://www.cancer.gov/
- NCRP (National Council on Radiation Protection & Measurements):
  http://www.ncrponline.org/
- NEMA (National Electrical Manufacturer's Association):
  http://www.nema.org/
- NMTCB (Nuclear Medicine Technology Certification Board):
  http://www.nmtcb.org/root/default.php
- North American Center for Continuing Medical Education:
  http://www.naccme.com/
- Nuclear Medicine Radiochemistry Society:
  http://www.radiochemistry.org/nuclearmedicine/
- Nuclear Medicine Technology Certification Board:
  http://www.nmtcb.org/root/default.php
- ODIA (Online Digital Imaging Academy):
  https://www.asrt.org/Applications/ODIA/
- Oxford Journals. Radiation Protection Dosimetry:
  http://rpd.oxfordjournals.org/content/
- Philips: http://www.healthcare.philips.com/
- RadiologyInfo.org: http://www.radiologyinfo.org/
- Radiological Society of North America: http://www.rsna.org/
- Radiopharmacy, Inc.: http://www.radiopharmacy.com/Newsletters.htm
- REMM (Radiation Emergency Medical Management):
  http://www.remm.nlm.gov/dictionary.htm
- Scintigraphy of the Pediatric Skeleton: http://www.medical-atlas.org/
- Siemens: http://www.medical.siemens.com/
- SNM (Society of Nuclear Medicine): http://www.snm.org/
- Societies of Nuclear Medicine of Latin America: http://www.alasbimnjournal.cl/
- UpToDate: http://www.uptodate.com/home/
- U.S. NRC Nuclear Regulatory Commission: http://www.nrc.gov/

Index

Printed by Publishers' Graphics LLC